Creating Lifetime Clients
How to WOW Your Customers for Life

FELICIA BROWN

Other Titles and Products by Felicia Brown

BOOKS

Free & Easy Ways to Promote Your Massage, Spa & Wellness Business:
Volume 1 – Getting Clients (& Keeping Them)
Reflections of My Heart: A Poetic Journey of Love, Life, Heartbreak & Healing
The Sunflower Princess: A Healing Fairy Tale
Contributing Author of *Thank God I…Volume 3*

E-BOOKS

How to Get New Clients
Getting Clients to Rebook
Upselling and Upgrading
Retailing for Massage, Spa & Salon Pros
Successful Event Planning Guide

HOME STUDY PROGRAMS

Smart Spa Marketing
Every Touch Marketing 6 Week Home Study Course
Every Touch Marketing 12 Week Intensive Home Study Course

CDs

Goal Setting: Create Success for Your Life and Business
Just Breathe: Guided Meditations for Inner Peace

ISBN: 0692567224
ISBN-13: 978-0692567227

DEDICATION

This book is dedicated to everyone who has supported me in my career as a massage therapist, most especially my own lifetime clients.

CONTENTS

BEFORE YOU START READING...

DOWNLOAD YOUR FREE RESOURCES!

Go to www.CreatingLifetimeClients.com and click on the tab for "Free Resources" to download the full-sized worksheets and exercises from the book – no promo code needed! You'll be able to print and use again and again as your business grows and changes. Download now so you can use as you read!

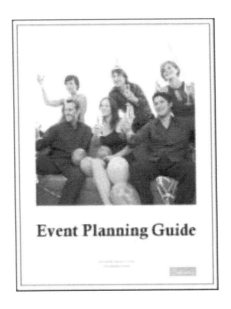

Event Planning Guide

As a bonus, I'm also including several additional special offers and discounts from massage and spa industry companies and organizations PLUS a **FREE Event Planning Guide** – perfect for organizing events and promotions!

Event Guide Description: Events created without careful planning are not likely to bring in many visitors, generate media interest or add extra sales. This detailed guide will help you prepare for many successful events in your business. Enjoy! fb

ACKNOWLEDGMENTS

There are so many people besides the author of a book who are a part of bringing it to life. I can't possibly name every person who has inspired or helped me in this particular endeavor, but I must single out a few specific individuals without whom what I have accomplished would not be possible.

My deepest gratitude to Eric Brown of Upside Brown for "right-on-time" mentoring, editing and overall support as well as the striking cover design and graphic help. I am so thankful you are a part of my world!

A big thank you also to:

~ Carol Houlihan Brown aka "Buttercup, the Book Doula" for helping me birth another baby book. Who knew joining a book club would lead to our friendship or other projects?!

~ My good friend, Shad Hills for the beautiful head shot/photograph for the back cover. I still love it!

~ Everyone who has invited me to teach and speak around the US, Canada and abroad over the last few years. It has been a blast! Special thanks also to my colleagues at Performance Health/Bon Vital, especially Lynda Solien-Wolfe and Marshall Daneke, for supporting me at so many of these events. I've had countless ideas and inspirations working with you.

~ My numerous conference buddies who have become dear friends: Angie Dubis; Joanna & Jesse Godwin; Tina Allen & Shad Hills; Tammy Moody; Dennis Buckley; Melanie Hayden & Scott Dartnall; Lorna Pascinato, Monica Forchelli & Robyn Green, Angie Patrick.

~ The readers of my blogs and books as well as my students and clients across the globe: It warms my heart to hear that something I said, wrote or did helped you somehow. Knowing I've touched your lives positively is why I write, teach and speak. Thank you!

~ My team and family at A to Zen: The commitment and love you bring to your work and clients is not only a joy to see but is a living affirmation of why A to Zen exists and flourishes. Your presence at A to Zen – whether brief or long-term – has added a special flavor to the "stone soup" of my career and life. I am grateful to each of you for putting your faith in me and helping create the best wellness spa in Greensboro, NC! You are LOVED!!

~ My former team and forever family at Stonehaven Massage & Spa: Our time together was a huge gift and restored my spirit in ways you may not realize. Together we accomplished a lot, and it is thrilling to see you all continue to blossom in new ways. I love and appreciate each of you for your role in my life, growth and healing. 🖥

~ A few special lifetime clients and friends – some who have been with me my entire career and others who immediately felt like we'd been connected for a lifetime: Seymour & Carol Levin, Len & Judy White, Irwin & Judy Smallwood, Frank & Nancy Brenner, Robin & Marti Tyler, Mary Marr & Freddy Johnson, Alan Irvin, Lou Pollock, Cindy Nordstrom, Fred Howes, and Janice Smith. Thank you for believing in me and making my job fun and rewarding every day!

~ My besties Susan Price, James Moore, Sharon Swift, Cathy & Bailey Jordan, Jed Corman, and the entire "old" Jaycee crew/MUSEPers.

Finally, thank you to my husband, David, for your continued love and unconditional support and acceptance of all that I am. I am so lucky to have you as my friend and partner in life.

Namaste, y'all.

Felicia

1 INTRODUCTION

Did you know there are only three ways to grow a business? I didn't either until a few years ago when I was assisting another instructor in a class on the topic. Prior to that moment, I thought there were countless ways to grow a business. For example, passing out my business cards wherever I go; doing free demonstrations or talks for community groups; running local advertisements; attending networking meetings - the list goes on and on, or so I thought.

However, regardless of how many different activities you're using to grow your business or sales, as my fellow educator said, there are only three primary methods to grow any business. The various activities I mentioned above are simply ways to accomplish of one, two or all three of those results.

Do you want to know what the three ways are? Drum roll please…..

1) **Attract more new clients**

2) **Get each client to come back again or more often**

3) **Sell more to each client with each visit or purchase.**

Sounds pretty simple, right?

The first strategy - **getting more new clients** – is the most obvious and what most people focus the bulk of their marketing efforts on. It can be accomplished in a variety of ways including the suggestions above as well as asking for referrals, providing giveaways, using social media or creating fun promotions. (Check out my first book, *Free & Easy Ways to Promote Your Massage, Spa & Wellness Business* to get some inexpensive ideas.)

On their own, paid advertising and grass-roots marketing can help you reach and become known to new clients. However there are quite a few people who will hesitate to try someone new, especially in the "touchy" area of personal services, because they are afraid of not getting what they want or need – and then feeling they wasted their time or money. To bridge the gap between their fear and your services, often an appealing – and sometimes costly - incentive is needed. While they can bring in large numbers of new clients, these incentives can wreak havoc on a small business if not planned and executed properly.

The point is, trying to find, reach and attract new clients often requires a large investment of some kind. In order to get a new client to spend money with a business which they have never tried, it can take quite a lot of time, money and effort. By retaining clients and turning them into lifetime clients, you'll reduce the costs of growing your business and put money back in your pocket where it belongs.

In fact, what may be more important than *getting new clients* is actually *keeping them*. As a business owner or massage professional, the second business building strategy you need to use is **retaining each client after their initial visit and encouraging them to do business with you more often.** Ideally, you want each new client to return for your products and services again and again – and hopefully, more frequently than once or twice a year.

2

Interestingly, a lot of professionals talk about their skills in client retention because they do see the same clients or customers over and over during the course of their long-term relationship. However, these same professionals fail to focus on ways to get their loyal, retained clients to see them or make purchases *more often*. Both are important in creating an ever-growing bottom line.

Finally, the third strategy for growing a business: **selling more to each client at each visit.** In an appointment based setting such as a spa, salon or massage clinic, this can be done fairly easily with service upgrades and upsells such as adding extra time onto a session, providing an additional service, or selling retail products. In a class or studio setting, this could involve offering private lessons or consultations, personal training, or other classes as well as suggesting products to enhance the class (or after-class) experience.

Even an upgraded membership or VIP plan can have an impact on your sales totals. And there are many different things you can do to get more activity from each client on each visit they make to your business. Regardless of how you do it, if you get your customers to spend a few more dollars whenever they are in your business, you are growing the revenue of your business without having to bring in more clients.

While all of these strategies are vital to growing a thriving business, this book will focus on the first and second topics: attracting new clients, and turning those new clients into lifetime clients who come back again and again, day after day, month after month, year after year. Clients who regularly rebook and repeat – and who I fondly call "bread and butter" clients – are the ones we really want to focus our efforts on finding and keeping.

Retaining clients helps you to save time, money, energy and effort. Studies show it takes five to ten times the amount of investment (time, money, energy and/or effort) to reach a new client and get them to try your business the first time than it does to get them to come back. In other words, once you've met and done a good job for someone, you've established the foundation of a "know, like and trust" factor which makes future business and sales much easier for them.

Client retention and long-term client relationships also create a more stable and predictable business. This is really important not just from a relationship standpoint or rapport but it's also important from an income forecasting perspective. When you can look at your schedule and know how many definite appointments you'll have each week, you can start to put together a financial picture of the revenue you'll bring in and better determine how to target future marketing efforts.

When you retain clients, you have a much better chance of giving your clients better results. By developing the rapport that comes in long-term relationships, clients will have more faith and trust in all you do. They'll be more likely to follow your suggestions for at-home care, additional treatments or visits, or outside referrals that will help them reach their goals. Thus, they are more likely to get better faster or feel better more often and that's going to make them happier clients.

It's important to understand that not all clients are going to be lifetime clients, nor would you want them to be. Before you begin seeking out ways to create long-term or lifetime relationships with your massage patrons, start by getting a clearer picture of your IDEAL clients. Here are three KEY things to consider:

1) Who will be best served by the services you offer

2) Which conditions and problems you excel in helping

3) What characteristics or qualities the people YOU enjoy working with posses

Once you determine your lifetime clients, you'll not only have a better idea of who you want to market to, but in turn should begin to see opportunities to reach out to them. Obviously, finding these folks is only half the job – you'll also have to meet their needs and get them to keep coming back. Strive to provide the results your ideal clients want and a high value along with a positive experience they can't get anywhere else. Doing so will help pave the way to a healthy long-term relationship.

In short, keeping clients for a lifetime isn't just about the money. It's also about giving clients what they need and want, so they feel happy with the relationship and themselves. Likewise, it's about creating career satisfaction, stability and joy for you, which, at least in my experience, translates into success for a lifetime.

Over the next few chapters, we'll dive in deeper and get you on your way to finding your own lifetime clients!

"Too often we underestimate the power of a touch, a smile, a kind word, a listening ear, an honest compliment, or the smallest act of caring, all of which have the potential to turn a life around."

— **Leo Buscaglia**

2 - ATTRACTING NEW CLIENTS

All businesses need to have a steady stream of new clients. No matter how good you are at what you do, client attrition is a fact of life due to life or job changes. People move, get sick, change careers, have a family, retire, and die. Their needs, goals and priorities shift with these changes, often leaving holes in our schedules and wallets. Thus most professionals need to bring new clients into their businesses as long as they are open.

Interestingly, over my years as an educator and marketing coach, one of the most common questions I heard was "What can I do to get more new clients, Felicia?"

I heard this from new professionals and seasoned solopreneurs alike. Some businesses get really caught up in focusing on bringing in first-time clients, maybe because it seems more exciting or logical to them. Though my standard rule of thumb is to focus 80% of marketing on current and past clients, and only 20% on reaching new ones, I know some owners pour most of their business development time, money, and energy into reaching new business. And it is good to find a variety ways to bring fresh faces into your business.

However, if your business is filled primarily with new clients and few who are returning patrons, you're working a lot harder than those with more established or repeat clients. (And, in truth, you probably need to take an honest look at the level of service, care and value you provide to determine why people aren't coming back.

> "To keep a customer demands as much skill as to win one."
>
> ~ American Proverb

The important thing to understand is this: getting people to come back and become repeat clients is much more cost-effective in the long run than only working with new clients. If you look at the amount of time, money, and energy it takes to bring someone new into your practice, it's much, much higher - five to ten times more, according to some studies - versus retaining the business of an existing client, it's really a no-brainer.

Why the drastically higher cost to reach new clients? There are a number of reasons, starting with the simple fact that they don't know about you until they know about you! As a complete unknown, you haven't even reached their Bottom of Mind Awareness (BOMA) when it comes to thinking about the services you offer.

In order to reach this subterranean level of awareness of your business, you could spend hundreds if not thousands of dollars on beautiful but expensive advertising with local magazines, newspapers, television and radio stations, and countless other venues – all to try and get potential new clients to notice you and what you offer. **This kind of marketing has a high out-of-pocket cost.**

You may also spend countless hours networking, offering free demonstrations, volunteering and educating the public to move beyond BOMA to MOMA (Middle of the Mind Awareness. These efforts definitely help add a know-like-and-trust factor more than any ad campaign ever could. However, they can still be a huge investment of your resources just to connect with potential clients in such a way that they actually feel comfortable enough to try you out. In other words, **this type of marketing has a high personal investment/time cost.**

Another option is providing some type significant incentive – perhaps a free upgrade, large discount or complimentary gift with their first visit – to get people to try you out. A notable example of this type of promotion is the various deals offered online by third-party companies. I won't refer to any specifically by name to avoid potential problems, but you likely know some of them.

These web-based companies promote personal services like massages, facials, spa treatments, hair and nail services, chiropractic care, acupuncture and a variety of athletic classes, memberships and services, for a very low price. The reason these promotions can be so successful is their connection to a large, targeted audience. Thus, the right offer has the potential to bring a large volume of fresh faces to a business. With the added appeal of no out-of-pocket or up-front cost to the business and a low risk to the consumers coming into the business, it seems like a match made in heaven!

Here's a basic overview of how these promotions generally work: The business owner determines what service, package, or product they want to promote on the site. The deal will often be structured for a savings of a little over 50% of the normal cost. (Various terms of the deal such as length of the offer, expiration dates, limitations or conditions, and even commission being negotiable.)

Assuming a typical massage or facial usually costs $80, and a potential customer only has to pay $39 for the service, it's almost too good for people to pass up. Sounds great, right? However, that offer costing the practitioner or business owner a portion of their regular earnings, both due to the discount as well as the share they pay to the promotional company. Depending on the company and deal, businesses are sometimes giving up 50% or more of what they would normally make on each new client who comes from the promotion. **This type of promotion has a high reduced-income cost.**

What often makes each of these types of "new client" promotions even more expensive is a lack of aiming them at the clients you are the most likely to retain.

SUMMARY

Remember, it's important to understand that not all clients are going to be lifetime clients, nor would you want them to be. Before you begin pouring your time, money and energy into trying to attract new clients, start building a clearer picture of your Ideal Lifetime Clients which we'll do in the next chapter.

3 - YOUR IDEAL LIFETIME CLIENTS

When you think about the term "lifetime clients," consider exactly who you'd be thrilled to see, talk to and do business with - week after week, month after month, year after year - for a lifetime. We've all had clients who we weren't really excited about seeing the first time, let alone again, because they weren't the right fit. That can make your days really long, can't it?

To get a clearer picture of who your ideal lifetime clients are, you need to really understand them. If we don't have a clear idea of who they are, then you're not going to do a very good job of attracting or keeping them.

Here are three KEY things to determine:

1) Who will be best served by the services you offer

2) Which conditions and problems you excel in helping

3) What characteristics or qualities the people YOU enjoy working with possess

It's important to get an overview of exactly who you are looking for as a lifetime client. Take a moment right now to make a list for each of these below. (Reminder: For a full-sized version of this and all other exercises in the book, go to www.CreatingLifetimeClients.com and click on the "Free Resources" tab to download.)

Who will be best served by the services I offer?

_____

_____

_____

_____

Which problems do I excel in helping or solving?

_____

_____

_____

_____

_____

What common characteristics or qualities do the people I enjoy working with possess?

_____

_____

_____

_____

_____

_____

From here, I want you to create a clear picture of what your ideal client looks like by creating a persona. A persona is basically a short paragraph that uses descriptive narrative to talk about your ideal client. I did this when I was seeking more of my own lifetime clients for my massage practice.

Felicia's Ideal Massage Client Description

My ideal clients are intelligent, genuinely nice, positive-minded people who enjoy life, learning new things and getting a great massage. They value getting weekly or monthly massages for stress reduction, pain relief and pure enjoyment. They are compassionate, understanding and loyal to those who meet their needs, win their trust and gain their friendship.

Though my ideal clients are generally healthy, they want to learn more about preventive care and improving their general wellness. They are moderately physically active to athletic (ex: running, golfing, tennis, Pilates and yoga) and appreciate how our work together plays a part in their overall fitness and well-being. They are also committed to taking an active role in their health and believe that getting regular massage is a vital part of that.

My ideal clients live within a five mile radius of my office and are between forty and eighty in age. They're well-established in their careers as executives, professionals, or entrepreneurs; comfortably retired; or home-makers and have flexible schedules, preferring appointments between 10 AM and 5 PM Monday through Friday or the occasional Saturday.

My ideal clients enjoy some conversation, are open-minded, and think of me as a professional and equal. They also appreciate "the good life" — travel, good food, wine, spas etc., but are down to earth, kind, friendly and generous. They refer freely, tip well, arrive on time and are a joy to work with in every session. Most of all they appreciate me as much as I appreciate them!

You'll notice that my description is very specific about what I was looking for in new clients. There was a method to my madness. As a therapist since 1994, some of my clients have been coming to me for more than 20 years. They're awesome people, and I want more people like them. I don't want just any random person coming to see me; I want to work with people that I love being around for another 20 years.

> **You are serving a customer, not a life sentence.**
> **Learn how to enjoy your work.**
>
> **~Laurie McIntosh**

And because I want to live a life I enjoy outside of work, I very specifically included details about the schedule I prefer. I'm not a morning person and don't want to be at my office at eight-thirty in the morning. Starting at ten o'clock gives me time to get up, work out – which is important to me - and then go to the office. At the end of the day, once you get much past 6 PM, I'm past my prime. I want to go home, have some dinner, and hang out with my dogs so starting with clients after five o'clock is a little too late for me.

Side note: When it comes to creating a schedule, in the beginning of practice or business, you probably need to be a little more flexible than my own description shows. As a well-established professional, I can dictate my schedule a little bit more than someone who is just starting out. In the beginning of my practice, I was available from 9:00 a.m. until 9:00 p.m., Monday through Friday, and from 9:00 a.m. to 6:00 p.m. on Saturday. I saw six clients a day, six days a week, and did so for several years. Now my needs and goals are different than they were at the start.

I want you to take action right now. Use the lists you made earlier about your ideal clients, as well as other ideas sparked by reading mine, to write as much of a Ideal Client Description as possible.

14

Think of as many characteristics, adjectives or qualities about your current or future favorite or ideal clients. Note: You may work with different groups or types of people, and that's perfectly okay. If so, you'll want to do this exercise for each different ideal lifetime client.

MY IDEAL LIFETIME CLIENT

_____

_____

_____

_____

_____

_____

_____

_____

_____

_____

_____

_____

_____

Your ideal client description(s) will most likely continue to evolve over time as your business does. I encourage you to continue to explore who you want to work with, and why, as well as who is most likely to use your products or services? You may also get more clarity on the problems your ideal clients want solved, or the feelings are they trying to achieve.

As you get to know your ideal clients better, you will also begin to notice other things they have in common with each other. In fact, if you want to be proactive, you could ask a few deeper questions of your ideal clients.

What do they do together? Where do they see each other? What neighborhood do they live in? What clubs do they belong to? Where are their kids in school? Which gym do they use?

Your ideal clients are unique. If you want to reach them, you have to find the special places that they go. Understanding where your ideal clients "live" and spend their time will give you quite a few clues as to where to find more people just like them.

A great example of this in my life: I have a lot of massage clients who enjoy drinking wine. Drinking wine and getting a massage don't usually go together during an actual appointment, but sipping some vino and relaxing certainly do. As well, those who enjoy the finer things in life like my ideal clients do, appreciate a robust Cabernet as much as a well-kneaded calf muscle. And in the case of some of my ideal patrons, a number of them happen to frequent the same wine bar and shop that I do, so it's been a good place to find even more like them. In the next chapter I'll share a bit more about how this has worked for me.

SUMMARY

Once you determine who you want to have as lifetime clients, you'll not only have a better idea of who you want to market to, but in turn will begin to see more opportunities to reach out to them. Obviously, finding these folks is only half the job. You'll also have to meet their needs and get them to come back. Strive to provide the results your ideal clients want and a high value along with a positive experience they can't get anywhere else. Doing so will help pave the way to a healthy long-term relationship.

4 - DOING WHAT YOU LOVE FOR A LIFETIME

If you are a massage therapist or healing arts provider like me, chances are you came into your profession because of a passion for making people feel better. In fact, if you are in any sort of a helping or healing profession, it's almost a given that you have a love of helping others.

> "Everyone has been made for some particular work, and the desire for that work has been put in every heart."
>
> ~ Rumi

However, you look at it, having a passion for what you do is an incredibly important factor in your long-term success. Thus it's time to get clearer on exactly what it is you really love to do. Let's start by just having a definition of exactly what passion is.

I think this quote from Brian Norris, author of *Escape Life Sucks Syndrome*, is just perfect for describing what passion is. He says, "Passion is a gift of the spirit combined with the totality of all the experiences we've lived through. It endows each of us with the power to live and communicate with unbridled enthusiasm." Further he says, "Passion enables us to overcome obstacles, both real and imagined, and to see the world as a place of infinite potential."

I want you to think about a couple of those sentiments, first of the idea of *unbridled enthusiasm*. Think about what that really means. A bridle is something that a horse uses, or I should say, the owner of a horse uses on a horse to keep it in control. So when something is unbridled, it's almost reckless, capable of running passionately and freely through the fields. Unbridled is about not being held back or restrained, in other words.

When it comes to creating and growing a successful business or practice, I think it's important to have a clear understanding of what you are or will be so excited about that you cannot contain it, something which causes you to burst with enthusiasm as you are waking up in the morning simply because you are thinking about doing it. That's real passion.

The other part of the quote I love is about overcoming obstacles. When you're really passionate about something, no mountain seems too tall. Sure mountains can be difficult to climb, but if something is truly important to you, you will climb a mountain, and probably quite a few, to get to the top. When you have passion it enables you to do things that you didn't know were possible. Trust me when I say, if you don't have passion, it can be a crippling handicap to your business and success.

I've owned several spas. The first one was extremely successful, not initially, but eventually. It took a huge investment of blood, sweat, and tears - and quite a bit of money - to reach the high level of success it did. Though there were plenty of problems getting there, because I had unbridled passion, nothing could hold me back. Every issue that got thrown in my way, I found a way around, over, or through it, because it was so important to me to bring that business into reality and make it successful. I was willing to go the distance, and do whatever it took, because I was so passionate about my vision. I wanted it in my bones and just knew that it was going to happen.

I remember talking to my landlord once about why he should give me three times the amount of space I had initially agreed to commit to. I didn't have the backing of a big investor or even a line of credit from a bank loan at the time. But because of my clear vision and level of unbridled passion, I convinced him to rent me the bigger space, and would figure out the financing later. He could feel my excitement and quickly got on board with me and my plans.

Several years later, after we had grown our sales to nearly two million dollars a year, I sold the spa because my passion for growing it (as well as the joy of owning it) was gone. I had taken it as far as I wanted and was very burned out. I never thought - at least at the moment I handed over my keys - I would go into the spa business again…but I did.

"The law of work seems unfair, but nothing can change it; the more enjoyment you get out of your work, the more money you will make."

~ Mark Twain

About three years after I sold my first spa, an opportunity arose for me to open another one. Unlike the first one which grew from a deep passion to create my own successful enterprise, at the second spa, the driving force was my desire to help a group of former employees. They were looking for a new opportunity and came to me because they'd enjoyed working for me before. Before the onslaught of phone class and requests for help from this group, I'd never seriously considered opening another spa. I was done. Yet something made me change my mind, call on my bank and plunge head-first into another venture.

For one, it looked like a great opportunity and chance to create something unique with people I enjoyed working with. It also looked like the spa would make a lot of money, so I thought, "Well, it's a good investment. I'll do it to help them and make some money." Unfortunately it didn't quite turn out the way I expected.

Looking back, I have to say, there were a number of issues that led to our downfall. One was the right timing, as we opened right before the economy kind of took a dive in 2008. Another was a team who was willing and able to do what it took to grow their part(s) of the business. Nearly everyone involved was an amazingly talented professional who – for good or bad – had only worked for me after my first spa was busy. None of them had the experience of growing a business from nothing into something nor the temperament to ride the waves of uncertainty that come with a new business. I did not see this as an issue until it was too late for it to matter.

However, the biggest thing missing from the business was me. My heart and the necessary passion drive for making the spa succeed was not there. Owning and running the spa day to day simply wasn't what I wanted. And so, after less than a year I decided to close that business, with some pretty harsh financial repercussions for doing so, I might add. But since my passion wasn't there, as soon as I made the decision to close it, I felt like a ton of bricks had been lifted off my shoulders.

The point is this: it doesn't matter how great of an opportunity something is, or how well everything seems to be lining up. What matters most is for your heart to be in whatever project you're taking on and that you're doing it for reasons which reward you as well as others. If you want to achieve true happiness and success, you have to go after things YOU want.

And, as difficult as being in business can be, YOU have to have the fire to make it happen, to get through, over, or around every obstacle you encounter, to have the unbridled enthusiasm I did. By ignoring this truth, I was treated to the most expensive lesson I've ever had in life and business. However, it was definitely one of the most valuable, which is why I share my story with you.

> "Your work is going to fill a large part of your life, and the only way to be truly satisfied is to do what you believe is great work. And the only way to do great work is to love what you do."
>
> ~ Steve Jobs

Now that you've read my story, I want you to think about yours a little bit. I invite you to turn on some soft music, maybe dim the lights, and do a short meditation exercise about your passion.

Begin by closing your eyes, taking a deep breath, and trying to empty your mind. Allow your wandering thoughts and questions to float away for a moment and just focus on the sensation of breathing in and out. Take a couple more deep breaths and relax your body into your chair. Feel your neck and shoulders release and settle into a place of calm and rest.

Bring your thoughts to something you get excited about at work. Let your mind wander and notice the first thing that comes to your mind. If you could do anything at all with your day, what would make you get excited in the morning and jump out of bed, raring to go? What would be so thrilling and engaging that you couldn't sleep or sit still just thinking about it? Picture this activity or scene in your mind and allow yourself to absorb or notice the feelings of excitement and anticipation.

If you can't quite picture what would have this affect on you, think instead about something – an event or activity – that brings you a deep level of satisfaction. What outcomes or results will cause you to look back on the day and feel really good about yourself?

Pause for a moment here and simply absorb the feeling of what it's like to feel happy, satisfied and excited by your work. Finish with another couple of deep breathes and open your eyes. While those images and feelings are fresh in your mind, take a few minutes write down the thoughts and inspirations you had during the meditation exercise.

MY PASSION

What makes you get excited about going to work?

_____

_____

_____

What makes you feel really satisfied, warm and fuzzy inside?

_____

_____

What do you most enjoy doing in your day?

_____

_____

What outcomes or results bring you the highest level of satisfaction and happiness at work?

_____

_____

You may continue to think of ideas after this journaling exercise, so keep writing your thoughts and ideas down. A couple of prompts you might use to get started include:

- ♥ _I am most passionate about doing, having, or being _____._

- ♥ _I am the most talented at providing _____ for my clients._

- ♥ _I love talking with my clients/colleagues about _____._

Remember to download the full sized worksheets and other goodies by going to www.CreatingLifetimeClients.com and clicking "Free Resources."

"It is an absolute human certainty that no one can know his own beauty or perceive a sense of his own worth until it has been reflected back to him in the mirror of another loving, caring human being."

— **John Joseph Powell**

5 FINDING IDEAL CLIENTS

Now that you've had a chance to really think about exactly WHO your ideal clients are we're going look at HOW to actually go out and find them. Targeting these people is of the utmost importance, especially if you want to retain them for the long haul. One of the most effective things you can do to find your ideal clients is to talk with existing ideal clients and ask them for referrals.

> **"The purpose of a business is to create a customer who creates customers."**
>
> ~ *Shiv Singh*

Client Referrals

If I could give you only one piece of advice about how to create a successful referral program, it would be this: **Make it simple.**

I've worked with almost all of my past coaching clients creating or improving their referral programs. All too often, what they've had in place or want to create is much too complicated! From requiring people to send multiple clients to get any sort of recognition to offering some type of sliding scale discount that changes with the number of referrals sent in, cumbersome referral programs like these are too complicated for clients to understand let alone participate in. Instead, I propose something very easy to explain and implement.

Some examples:

- *Refer a new client and save $5 on your next facial.*

- *Invite a friend to try us out! After they come in, you'll receive credit for a 15 minute massage upgrade.*

- *Get a free sauna session with every successful new student referral to our Monthly Tai Chi program.*

Just as with other kinds of promotions, you may also want to extend a special offer to the person being referred by your current client. Since this person knows you through association, it need not be as big of an incentive as you might give to someone who has no connection whatsoever. (Note: *As in all areas of business, please be familiar with the laws regarding referrals as they relate to your profession and area.*)

How to use new client referral cards and certificates:

- Give at least three to every client you see
- Give with or in place of your business card at networking events
- Pass out anywhere you interact with a sales person or cashier
- Send them out in your Christmas/holiday cards
- Include them with retail or gift certificate purchases
- Hand them out with appointment reminder cards
- Give them to clients to send out in their holiday cards

- Send them to businesses you patronize to put in employee paychecks or pass out to their clients

- Ask other small businesses to put a stack at their cash register or wherever they post info from other businesses

- Leave as an additional tip when you eat out

- Enclose in birthday cards to your friends

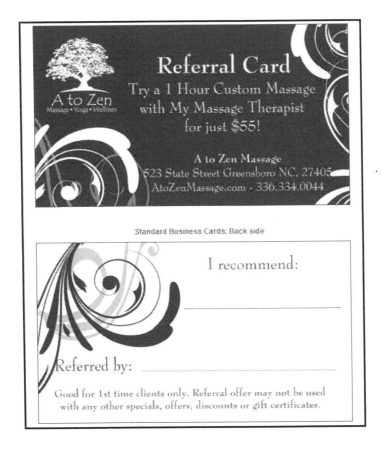

The card above is actually what we currently use in my own business. For more details on referrals <u>and</u> the details of the most successful referral promotions I've done so far, check out my book *Free &*

Easy Ways to Promote Your Massage, Spa & Wellness Business at Spalutions.com or EveryTouchMarketing.com.

Professional Referral Partners

If you've taken the time to learn about who your ideal clients are, you've no doubt discovered a few common places, people or activities that many of them connect with or engage in regularly.

> "Loyal customers, they don't just come back, they don't simply recommend you, they insist that their friends do business with you."
>
> ~ *Chip Bell*

For example, a number of my ideal clients really enjoy drinking wine, as do I. At the end of the last chapter, I mentioned a quaint wine shop which has served double duty for me as a place to unwind while at the same time reaching some of my ideal clients. Over the years, I've been to that wine shop with some friends who are also clients. My friends, being who they are, bragged about what a great massage therapist I was, and soon the owners – as well as a few other friends - were on my table or seeing other therapists in my office. Both owners became regular clients and purchase packages of prepaid massage on a regular basis.

They also refer others: People who are in the wine shop relaxing at the end of the day, maybe talking about what a stressful week they've had or a headache that just won't go away. The owners pay individual attention to their patrons, and being the kind of people that want to meet their clients' needs, offer a variety of solutions. Since drinking wine isn't going to eradicate all the pain and stress people have, they often suggest massage. Although we've never put any specific program in place outside of our standard referral program, we have done a few special promotions here and there and value this relationship because of the targeted reach they have with our ideal clients.

Another referral partner I've worked with is a local physical therapy office. One of the PTs sent me a letter introducing himself and the business. Essentially they wanted to get to know my business as they were searching for a massage therapy practice to send some of their PT patients to for relaxation and pain relief.

I paid them a visit, tried out their services (dry needling in particular), and got to know the professionals in the practice. I also invited each of their staff members to come try us out (see *New Client Post Card* on the next page) with a complimentary 30 Minute Massage Upgrade. They in turn came in for their massages, some on their own, and others with their spouses. It was a great fit for both businesses, and soon the referrals began to flow in both directions!

Some businesses that fall into this area might not be a direct referral partner as these two have, but they might be able to work with you in some other kind of a way. An example of this might be a chiropractor, that doesn't have a massage therapist on staff. Maybe they're not quite ready to refer business to an outside massage therapist, but they'd be willing to do an event with one.

Ideal situations could be a program or lecture in which you both present topics of interest to the same audience. Or perhaps you each give out coupons or initial consultation certificates while sharing a booth at a trade show. (See the next page for a sample coupon I use in situations like this.)

Another example could be a real estate broker because boy, they're stressed out, aren't they? They're running all the time, working nights and weekends, dealing with demanding homeowners and all kinds of details that you don't even want to know about that go into real estate. But they're also a gateway to other ideal clients, particularly if they're serving a neighborhood where your ideal clients live. Perhaps you can connect with them to provide gifts for them to share with new homeowners or for those who refer potential home buyers and sellers to them.

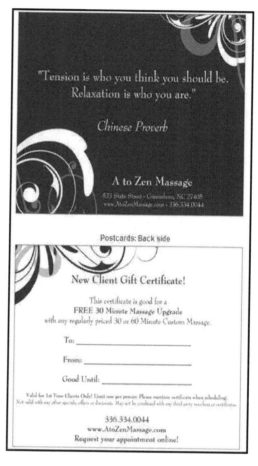

A similar example: One gentleman I worked with was an insurance agent who had a lot of real estate brokers as his clients. To say thank you to the brokers in largest customer's firm, he paid for an afternoon of chair massage in the broker's office. In turn, we introduced ourselves to the brokers and let them know how we could help them help their own businesses.

Let's take time now to get clear on WHERE to find your ideal clients so you can better connect with IDEAL referral partners.

WHERE ARE MY IDEAL CLIENTS?

What neighborhood(s) do your ideal clients live or work in?

_____

_____

What businesses are in that neighborhood(s) that could be a good referral partner? Start with those in which you already know someone or there is an obvious connection between your services/products.

_____

_____

_____

What schools do they or their children attend?

_____

_____

What clubs or organization(s) do they belong to?

_____

_____

What charities or causes do they contribute to or support?

_____

_____

What other stores(s) do your ideal clients shop in?

_____

_____

What gym or sporting facilities do they use or belong to?

_____

_____

What sports do they (or their kids) watch or participate in?

_____

_____

_____

What other professionals have you heard them mention? (Think personal trainer, tailor, chiropractor, counselor, etc.)

_____

_____

_____

_____

As you fill in the blanks, you may want to go back to your ideal client description and add a few more details to it.

Vendor Referrals

Something you might not have thought of in terms of targeting ideal clients is the products that they use, and working with product companies which these people love and recognize. When people know, like and trust a product for the results it gets, they will seek it out again and put some of that confidence in the providers that use them.

A great example of this kind of product - and one I use in my wellness spa - is Biofreeze®. Biofreeze® is a great topical pain reliever, and has a very recognizable name. In fact, it seems people in pain will go out of their way to find it. Perhaps it was recommended to them in the past by a former health professional or a friend who has used it. Regardless, it's a name that stays in their mind. Thankfully, Biofreeze has a Product Locator feature on their website which can help direct those seeking it to the various practitioners and businesses that carry it.

(Go to www.Biofreeze.com/whereToBuy.aspx to find professionals in your area that carry it. To become listed as a practitioner who sells Biofreeze, go to http://www.biofreeze.com/page/en/online.aspx).

Many product lines do this, especially in the spa, skin and salon world. If you happen to be the one that carries a hard-to-get or an in-demand line or product, and particularly if that product is something that serves your ideal clients, getting listed on the brand's locator service could very well become a source of new and ideal client referrals.

Advertising for Ideal Clients

Of course, you can look at traditional paid advertising as a means of reaching your ideal clients. In one of the neighborhoods where my ideal clients live, there's a new magazine written just for homeowners. Though it's fairly expensive to do so, each month I advertise. I know my ad is being seen by exactly who I want to see it. That being said, whatever money you do decide to spend in this area should be very carefully considered.

> "The aim of marketing is to know and understand the customer so well the product or service fits him and sells itself."
>
> ~ *Peter Drucker*

Besides print media, there are countless places to advertise, from magazines, television and radio to individual events, sponsorships, printed and online coupons, and so many other things. However, as a general rule, I believe in finding ways to market without spending lots and lots of dollars for advertising. In fact, there are plenty of other things that you could do.

You could look for athletic events and races if you happen to be looking for athletes; causes and charities if you're looking for a good-hearted population; or if you want to target people with a certain condition, you might seek out support groups or physicians that cater to those issues.

Look back at the lists you made earlier in the chapter and use your answers as a guide for potential advertising and marketing vehicles. Use mine on the next page as a guideline to help direct your own ads and other marketing ventures.

EXAMPLE: WHERE FELICIA'S IDEAL CLIENTS ARE

What neighborhood(s) do your ideal clients live or work in?
Irving Park – *Irving Park Magazine; direct mail*

What businesses are in that neighborhood(s) that could be a good referral partner? Start with those in which you already know someone or where there is an obvious connection between your services/products.)

Kallos Hair Salon – *networking for wedding packages*
State Street Jeweler – *gift certificate for purchases over $500*
Kriegsman Furs – *gift certificate for purchases over $500*
Dance Studio – *networking with instructors*
State Street Shoppes – *Facebook posts, shared ads in local paper*

What schools do they or their children attend?
St. Pius – *advertise in parents' news letter, sponsor sports team*
Greensboro Day School – *sponsor alumni events*

What clubs or organization(s) do they belong to?
Greensboro Country Club – *massage therapist on staff*

What charities or causes do they contribute to or support?

Hospice – *sponsor Triathlon for Hospice; attend Hospice health fairs*

Symphony Guild – *advertise in seasonal newsletter*

What other store(s) do your ideal clients shop in?

EarthFare – *community bulletin board*

What gym or sporting facilities do they use or belong to?

The Club – *have massage, spa and salon on-site*

What sports do they (or their kids) watch or participate in?

Yoga – *offer free chair massage after classes at Lululemon*

Running – *sponsor local running events, join running club*

Golf – *sponsor tees at local tournaments, get involved in First Tee of the Triad (local golf organization and charity)*

What other professionals have you heard them mention?
(Ex. personal trainer, tailor, chiropractor, counselor, etc.)

Joey M. (Personal Trainer) – *networked in the past, has a massage therapist on-site now*

Samantha J. (Esthetician) – *discussed trade but potential conflict of interest due to our esthetician tenant*

Grace P (Pilates Instructor) – *set up a referral partnership*

Dr. Byron B (plastic surgeon) – *offer complimentary services to office staff; suggest corporate pricing for volume purchases of services for client gifts*

SUMMARY

Whatever types of promotions you decide to do, be looking for your ideal clients wherever they happen to be. Get started on building those referrals and connections with the people who serve your ideal clients. It's probably going to take a little bit of research on your part, but will be a significant step to build referrals for your ideal clients – and totally worth the effort!

"If I could touch anything in the world right now, it would be your heart. I want to take that piece of you and keep it with me."

— **Jessica Verday**, **The Haunted**

6 CREATING EXPERIENCES OF A LIFETIME

In **Free & Easy Ways to Promote Your Massage, Spa & Wellness Business**, I wrote "marketing is everything that 'touches' a client and makes them want to come to you the first time, the next time, or perhaps the last time." It's every interaction you have with a client, whether it's you personally, or it's your business card, or your voicemail, or your website or whatever.

When we're talking about attracting and keeping lifetime clients, it's important for us to understand why they come to us in the first place. A lot of people think they have a definition of why people come in and get massage or why they want facials, or why they come to a spa, but essentially it's a combination of reasons.

It could be they want to improve their health and well-being, decrease their pain and discomfort, or escape from stress. Perhaps they want to be restored and renewed, have some peace and quiet, and take a little mini vacation. In the case of skin-care, clients may have specific beauty or aging concerns they're looking to address. Or on the wellness side, they may want to feel better or live a healthier lifestyle.

I want you to think about your favorite spa, massage, or other wellness service experience ever. It could be a massage experience or your favorite facial. Take a moment to answer these three questions:

What exactly made the experience so special?

_____

_____

What stands out in your mind about the experience?

_____

_____

Why did you want to go back again?

_____

_____

Chances are good that your favorite experience stood out in your mind because the business and the professionals in it provided a good combination of the RESULTS you wanted (relaxation, pampering, pain relief, etc.) along with an outstanding experience that made you FEEL something you don't get in other businesses (understood, appreciated, cared for, safe, respected, heard, etc.).

Whatever the winning combination was, it didn't happen by accident and was most likely the result of an attentive and skilled professional or team.

Unfortunately, as often as I've asked this question in classes around the US and Canada, very few people are able to share examples of a perfect, wonderful or even simply memorable positive experiences in massage, day spa or salon businesses and settings. Why?

If we haven't communicated with clients properly about their needs and wants – as well as the general procedures for their appointments

- the experience can quite easily become confusing, scary, overwhelming and even disappointing. How would you feel if you didn't know you had to get undressed for your first massage, or that you shouldn't shave for a week or two before you had a bikini wax?

These types of surprises can make a visit to the spa, salon or wellness center much less enjoyable and effective than what the client had hoped for. Some people end up feeling frustrated or angry. Others think the price they paid - no matter what it was - was too expensive or not a good value. The bottom line is they end up feeling stressed and unhappy as a result of us not paying attention to or anticipating their needs. As a result, we lose their business and loyalty before we had a real chance to earn it.

Starting off Right

As caring professionals seeking to cultivate rapport and long-term relationships with our clients, we want to make sure whenever possible to meet the clients' needs and deliver an unforgettably positive experience. To do this and get the clients to not only come back but to become lifetime devotees of our services, we must begin by anticipating each client's needs and wants before they even arise.

For example, since my office can be difficult to find, I email new clients specific, descriptive directions to the office as soon as they book their appointment. To save time, I also send a link to my website where they can download and print the appropriate client intake forms and fill out before their appointment. I also send email appointment reminders to all clients about 48 hours before the appointment. They know they can count on the reminder so they're not unexpectedly missing an appointment. These are now all automated via our scheduling software, but can be done manually as well.

Another example: We keep robes on the back of the doors of our treatment rooms. If a client needs to get up in the middle of their session for any reason, they won't have to get dressed again.

31+ Points of Contact in a Massage, Spa or Wellness Business

Before the Appointment

1 – Website, Menu & Business Cards

2 – PR, Marketing & Advertising

3 – Logo and Image

4 – Reputation & Buzz (including online reviews)

5 – Exterior Appearance & Signage

6 – Location/Directions, Ease of Access & Parking

7 - Phone & Scheduling

8 – Greeting & Welcome

Inside the Business

9 – Waiting and Retail Areas

10 - Products sold & used

11 - Tour of Facility/Menu

12 - Explanation of Services

13 – Attitude of and Greeting by Professional/Staff

14 – Treatment Room(s)

15 –The Service Itself

16 –What Happens in the Service

After the Appointment

17 – Ending the session

18 – Paying the bill

19 –Specials/rewards/programs

20 – An invitation to return/rebooking

21 – Farewell and thank you

22 – Post-Visit Marketing

- Birthday card

- Thank you note

- Referral discount

- Follow up calls

- Email updates

General Operations

23 – Facility in good repair

24 – Clean restrooms and locker rooms

25 – Amenities available

- Water/Tea

- Snacks/Mints

- Robes/slippers

- Lockers

- Steam/sauna/whirlpool

- Wi-Fi

26 – Flow of visit

27 – Uniforms and appearance of staff

28 – Extra touches

- Candles

- Art

- Flowers

- Table treats

Memories that last

29 – Music type & noise levels

30 – Scents and aromas

31 - New client gifts

Clearly, there are many details and "touches" that go into gaining a client's lifetime loyalty. Dropping the ball on any one of them can create the potential for making a negative impression and losing that person's future business and referrals.

How do you think you are doing in each of these areas? Are you brave enough to find out by asking your clients? Go to www.CreatingLifetimeClients.com to download a full-sized resource handout which includes the **31 Points of Client Contact** as well as the following survey. A full sized version/download is available in the book's free online resources at www.CreatingLifetimeClients.com).

Client Survey

Thank you for taking this short survey. Please circle as many choices as apply for each question. What do you like most about my business?

- ♥ Appointment availability
- ♥ Hours/schedule
- ♥ Prices
- ♥ Services available
- ♥ Location/area
- ♥ Décor /setting
- ♥ Products used
- ♥ Products sold
- ♥ Quality/value
- ♥ Prompt service
- ♥ Online gift certificates
- ♥ Online scheduling
- ♥ Payment options available
- ♥ Communication methods available
- ♥ Therapist Experience
- ♥ Other (fill in below)
- ♥ _____

Comments:

_____

_____

What do you like least (or feel needs improvement) about my business?

- ♥ Appointment availability
- ♥ Hours/schedule
- ♥ Prices
- ♥ Services available
- ♥ Location/area

- ♥ Décor /setting
- ♥ Products used
- ♥ Products sold
- ♥ Quality/value
- ♥ Prompt service
- ♥ Online gift certificates
- ♥ Online scheduling
- ♥ Payment options available
- ♥ Communication methods available
- ♥ Therapist Experience
- ♥ Other (fill in below)

_____

Comments:

_____

_____

What are your preferred communication methods from me/ABC Spa?
- ♥ Email
- ♥ Phone Call
- ♥ Text message
- ♥ Social Media postings
- ♥ Direct mail
- ♥ Other _____

Which – if any – of the following do you use on a regular basis?

- ♥ Facebook
- ♥ Twitter
- ♥ Linked In
- ♥ Pinterest
- ♥ Yelp
- ♥ Instagram
- ♥ Read blogs

♥ Check email

What would you be most interested in learning about via events, newsletters, and social media channels/pages? Circle all that apply.

*self care to do at home
*health and wellness tips
*weight loss/diet tips
*beauty/skin care tips
*anti-aging
*Information about other services, products
*Organic/green issues, causes and products
*Other: _____

Are you comfortable referring others to me/ABC Spa? Why or why not?

_____
_____
_____

If you are generally happy with my services, products and business, can you share a short comment or testimonial about your experience here and what you enjoy most about my business/services?

_____
_____
_____

May we use your comments as a part of our marketing? YES   NO

May we include your name with your comments? YES   NO

Name (Optional): _____

Preferred email address (Optional): _____

Preferred phone contact (Optional): _____

Special Touches

Beyond the obvious necessities of business operations, there are a lot of small and subtle touches that can make an indelible impression on the mind and heart. The following are a few examples of special touches from my wellness spa that have helped bond the relationships I have with some of my long-time regulars:

I do whatever I can to make each of my clients feel special and cared for, especially in ways which matter to them. One of my ideal clients, Judy, adores Wintergreen Lifesavers and I make it a point to always have plenty on hand for her. When I first realized Judy loved those Lifesavers, I started decorating the table with them every time she came in. Before every appointment, I (and any other therapist she sees at the spa) will decorate the table in a different design of lifesavers every time she comes in. We do it because Judy loves them so much and she gets a kick out of the effort we make. She has earned the nickname "the Lifesaver Lady" and adores them as a special treat.

> **"The first step in exceeding your customer's expectations is to know those expectations."**
>
> **~ Roy H. Williams**

Let me share a quick story about Judy to illustrate just how important the little things are: Judy has been coming in to my various businesses for massage approximately once a month for over 20 years. In addition to being a great client, she's also one of those people who just lights up the door when she comes in. She often tells me at the end of a massage, "Oh Felicia, that was an A plus-plus!"

I have to tell you, that's what I really love about doing massage – the positive feedback and instant gratification of praise I get for a job well done. In fact, that regular positive affirmation is part of what

46

makes Judy one of my ideal clients. It's a little bit embarrassing to admit part of why I'm still passionate about this business is hearing when I do something well, but it's totally true.

One day a few years ago, Judy came in to get her massage and said to me, "Oh Felicia, I have been looking forward to this massage all day long, and there are three reasons."

"Wow, I can't wait to hear them," I said, waiting with breathless anticipation. I'm excited and primed about the forthcoming compliments about my work and how great I am -- silly, but true.

So she says, "Number one, I knew you'd have a cold bottle of water waiting for me. I've been on the go and so thirsty all day long. I couldn't wait to come in and drink some of it."

I thought, "Okay, water, there's water on the table for every client and that doesn't seem so special. But alright, Judy likes the water! That's good to know. Now she's going to talk about how great I am."

Next she says, "Number two, oh Felicia, I love those positive thought cards that you put on the table. They are my favorite, and I couldn't wait to see what mine was going to say."

Still, she said nothing about the massage. But I'm thinking, "Awesome. She loves the water and the positive thought card. The next compliment's going to be about me!"

So I'm waiting, you know, on pins and needles when Judy says, "Number three. I couldn't wait to get my Lifesavers. I've got three of them in my mouth right now!"

Stunned, I asked, "That's great, Judy. Was the massage even part of what you were looking forward to?"

With a shrug she replied, "Oh yeah, that too," before she walked into the massage room and shut the door.

The point of this story is how the little things made Judy so excited to come in and see me for a massage. Who would think someone with has tons of stress and lots of aches and pains would be more excited to tell me about her anticipation of getting a bottle of water, card and Lifesavers than the massage? I certainly didn't and was admittedly a little bit disappointed I didn't get the compliment I was craving. However, I did get some really valuable insights!

> **"Revolve your world around the customer and more customers will revolve around you."**
> **~ Heather Williams**

I have another client who loves Tootsie Rolls, but not the miniature ones we have in the spa for the rest of the clients. Just for her, I keep a bag of the regular sized candies in my treatment room and make sure to put a couple on the table before each of her appointments.

Not all clients love candy, but everyone has their preferences about what they like during a massage - and I keep detailed notes about them. Some of my clients like hot towels and aromatherapy. Others prefer a cool room and no blanket when they come in. Some folks like a bolster under their feet and some like a pillow. Remembering these extras and providing clients with what suits them best helps me to set myself apart from other therapists. It's often the little things that turn people into lifetime clients!

Now you might be saying, "Gosh Felicia, why do I want to treat some clients differently? Isn't it better, to treat all of my clients well but the same?"

Yes and no. You want to cater to all your lifetime clients at the same level but in individual ways whenever possible. When you employ relationship-based thinking about current and potential lifetime clients versus appointment-based thinking for one-time or occasional clients, you will begin to act a little bit differently. So yes, I do want you to employ this high level of individualized care with all of your clients. When you connect with each person on a deeper level while meeting their needs, you'll exceed their expectations and they will likely want to see no one but you.

Through my interactions and observations, I know without a doubt Judy and the rest of my ideal and regular clients have specific things which keep them coming back as loyal clients besides my massage abilities. It isn't just about technical skills. It's important to understand that, because many service professionals think the reason our clients come to us, our ideal clients even, is because of the service we offer. And true, that is a part of it. We are professionals, and I'm sure each of you does an amazing job with your hands-on skills and taking care of your clients' aches, pains, stress and tension. But the truth is that it's often the little things – those tiny details that other people miss - that really cement their relationship with you for the long term.

Consistency and Follow Up

It's easy to impress someone once, but can you keep up the quality after the first visit? When we're talking about client retention, especially with lifetime clients, it's not just about making a great impression the first time. It's about continuing that level of care day in and day out, week after week, so that every time that person sees you they feel special.

Unfortunately, it's very easy to become complacent with people once you've won them over. (Look at the majority of marriages and you'll see what I mean.) Thus, I encourage you to think about how you can continue to touch your clients in different and unexpected ways, not just on your table or during your service, but throughout your business.

Something I use in my office is these positive or healing thought cards. In the past I used cards made by other authors like Louise Hay and Wayne Dyer, but I decided to make my own a few years ago. Each one has a photograph or illustration on one side and a positive thought, affirmation or a quote on the other. When my clients come in, there's a card waiting for them on the table. It's something different that sets me apart and something that people notice. The comment that I get most often is "Wow, did you pick this out for me? It really spoke to me!" When I tell people I didn't pick it out, I just put a card on the table randomly, they're often amazed with how it fits exactly with what they needed that day.

> "Every contact we have with a customer influences whether or not they'll come back. We have to be great every time or we'll lose them."
>
> ~ *Kevin Stirtz*

What sometimes touches people even more is the fact that I tell them they can keep the card when they leave. They love that it's not just something they have to try and remember but it's instead can take out the door with them as a tangible reminder of their massage and our time together.

****

You can see samples from each card deck I've created on the following pages. Most are available for purchase at www.Spalutions.com and www.EveryTouchMarketing.com.

50

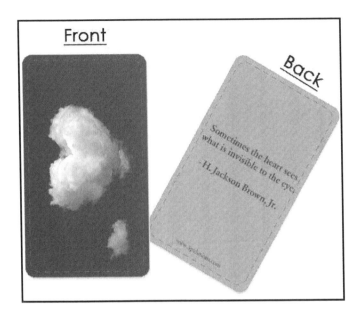

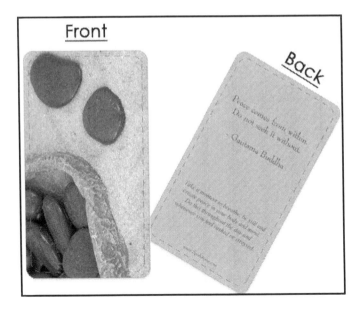

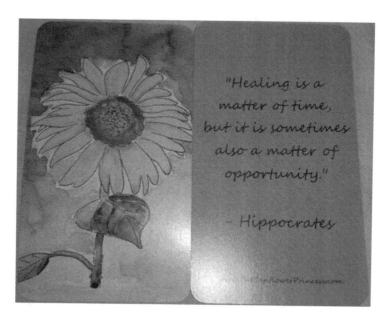

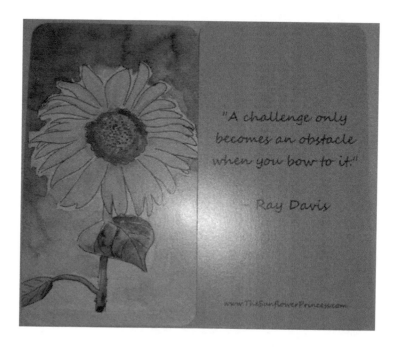

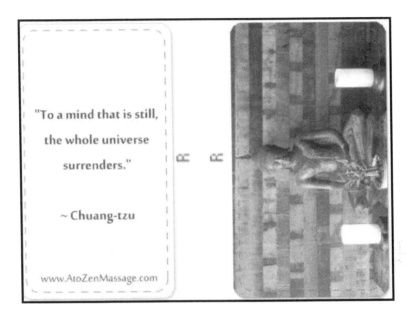

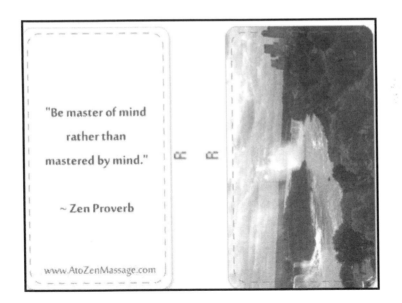

Some other things we do to make clients feel special and valued:

- Send every new client a hand written thank you note after the first visit.

- Provide a new client gift, currently an organic soap bar.

- Send an email asking how their first experience was – from me – with an invitation to share any comments or feedback with me directly as well as to write a review.

- Send a birthday postcard AND a birthday email.

- Send emails after they have not been in for 6 weeks and 12 weeks.

- Provide a Valentine's Day gift for every client in February.

- Send ongoing emails about specials, new services, healthy living tips and our team.

- Call regular clients with open appointments and cancellations.

The last suggestion of calling clients is an art which seems to be falling by the wayside. If this type of client interaction makes you nervous, why not write down a script or checklist of what you plan to say? Then practice your dialogue before the call. When you finally get up the nerve to call the first person, take a deep breath, relax and remind yourself that your intention is to let clients know that you miss and care about them, as well as to share an offer that will help them save money and take care of themselves.

Here's a quick example of what I might say:

"Hi _____. It's Felicia from A to Zen. It's been a while since you were last in and we miss seeing you here. How've you been?"

Wait for client response

"I'd like to give you a special offer to come in this week/month for another facial. The welcome back offer is your choice of a Deluxe facial for the price of a Standard Facial session OR a 15% off any service. Which would you prefer?"

Make sure to have a list of times ready that might appeal to those you call based on past visits and your availability. Put a friendly tone in your voice and smile while you are talking. Remind yourself that even if they don't book, you are in no worse shape business-wise than you were before you made the call. But if you don't follow up with those who have expressed an interest in working with you - past, present or future - they may never call (again) on their own. And that's a sure way to fail in any business.

Right now I want you to take action and I want you to write down at least three things you can do to connect with your ideal clients on a deeper level and three ways you can maintain that connection through follow ups. I've given you plenty of ideas that I use in my spa and I'm sure you have others of your own.

How I Plan to Connect on a Deeper Level

_____

_____

_____

_____

How I Plan to Follow Up Consistently

_____

_____

_____

_____

Walt Disney said, "Do what you do so well that they will want to see it again and bring their friends." If you think about the success of Disneyland and Disney World you know he followed this to a "T." You too, can do some amazing things in your business to help bring clients in the first time, the next time, and again and again. Those simple touches and ways you connect, that you listen to your clients and really give them an experience they can't have with anyone else, and by knowing exactly who those people are, that they're going to treasure and love those experiences, the ones that utilize your passion and talents, you're absolutely going to be a success.

SUMMARY
No matter what your area of expertise, there are a multitude of businesses in the world and countless places people can go to spend their money and their time on. When you're trying to attract lifetime clients to your business, you need to be ready to touch or reach them in a way they're not getting anywhere else, especially when someone has pain, or is struggling, or even just really stressed out. If you do something that makes them stop, and think, and reflect, it really makes an impact. If you are making time to connect with people, to serve the needs they tell you about, along with some that they don't even know they have, they will feel really special and want to come back and see you again and again, for a very long time.

7 GETTING IDEAL CLIENTS TO RETURN

It should be clear by now that in order to get a new client to risk spending time and money with you - an unknown business or professional - can take quite a lot of time, money and effort. However, once they've tried your business the first time, you've established a "know, like and trust" factor, and perhaps connected with them on a deeper level. Future visits will seem much less risky. As a bonus, keeping new clients in your business helps you save the time, money, energy and effort you've invested.

Besides reducing your investment, long-term client retention creates stronger rapport and stability with each client who returns. Previously, you may not have given much thought regarding the impact on healing, transformation or progress which comes with client retention, but you might be surprised by the things that can happen as a client gets to know, like and trust you. First of all, the longer you do business with someone, the more they're going to feel comfortable with you. At each and every session, they're going to feel more relaxed and confident in your abilities. As a result, they're going to have better results, feel better about coming to see you, and be more likely to send you business, all making your job easier.

As for you as a professional or practitioner, this level of comfort and trust means you're going to enjoy your job more as well. Just think about the difference of meeting or working with someone brand new for the first time. There is a level of nervousness which goes along with that kind of scenario as well as thoughts like, "Oh, I have to prove myself and win this person over." This type of nerve-wracking interaction is a lot different than a day when you see familiar faces crossing your door all day long, isn't it?

Imagine waking up to see your appointment calendar and... *ahhh*...breathing a sigh of relief because you've already passed the initial "new client" phase with the folks you have scheduled.

"Oh, what an awesome day it's going to be! Joe is coming in at 10 AM and he is so funny. Then I get to see Mary at 11:30. She has such a calming personality. I can't wait to find out if the stretches I gave her for the calf cramps helped. And I really like working with Jennifer. I wonder how her race went this weekend?!"

Days and clients like these are part of what makes our careers really rewarding, especially if you're like me and want to know you're making a difference in other's lives. By contrast, when you are working with all new clients, every day and session is a complete mystery. Sure, you can have some amazing and gratifying experiences with brand new clients, hopefully they can too. However, when you have clients you see on an ongoing basis, you get to see the difference your work or services have made in others lives, which often provides a deeper level of professional satisfaction and reward.

As a client returns again and again, you'll develop a stronger level of trust and rapport. Typically, as the relationship grows, they'll achieve better, more consistent results, regardless of what type of work you do. Because they get better faster or feel better more often, they will be happier than if they were going a variety of places for the same service. They'll feel good about the choices they've made and so will you.

Clearly, retaining clients for the short-term or a lifetime is not purely about the money; it's also about creating a really satisfying life for yourself as a practitioner. Relationships which have depth of rapport, connection, trust and comfort between you and your clients are mutually beneficial. The more comfortable you are in treating them, the more you're able to really give from your heart and the more they're actually able to receive it in the deepest way possible.

> "You don't earn loyalty in a day.
> You earn loyalty day-by-day."
>
> ~ Jeffrey Gitomer

Client retention and satisfaction also leads to increased services and revenue, something anyone in business should want. If you're in business for yourself and money isn't important to you, you might need to look at why you feel that way. Unless you're already independently wealthy, it's important for a business to keep growing in profitability and other rewards.

What this means from a business standpoint is the better the relationships and retention you have, the more this translates into increased services or classes as well as better retail sales, all of which will increase your revenue (and probably your tips as well if you're in a business where you get tipped.) Likewise, your clients are happier because they're getting what they want and feel that they're at home in a way. That's something that a first-time client is almost never going to experience.

While client retention isn't just about the return on an investment, it can be helpful from an income forecasting perspective. As you develop a loyal, regular and more predictable clientele, you will notice patterns and trends in your schedule. By knowing, at least in part, who is likely to come in each week or month, you can start to put together a picture of your projected income and determine where you need to do some extra marketing or follow up.

Hopefully, you're starting to say "Wow! Client retention isn't just about not having to find so many new people to do business with. It's about really getting the best results possible for each client and having the best practice I can."

As a massage therapist in practice for over twenty years, many of my existing clients have been with me almost the whole time I've been in practice. When they come in, it's like seeing a member of the family and there's a huge comfort in that. It's also large part of why I'm still practicing after all this time. I love my clients and truly enjoy seeing them when they come in the door. Keep that in mind as decide whether to spend most of your marketing efforts on getting new clients or retaining old ones.

How to Make It Happen

If you're serious about client retention versus having mostly new clients, then it's time to move beyond a transaction or appointment-based mentality into a lifetime client mentality. So, think for a moment if you will, about the last time you had an appointment that was "just a brow wax, or "only a thirty-minute massage," or "a Groupon." Most of us have all at some point been guilty of minimizing the importance and impact of these seemingly small or unpromising sessions, I promise you. So I want you to ask yourself honestly, if you treat a new client with a shorter or less expensive appointment, or even a special occasion client, differently than someone who is receiving a regularly priced service? Do you give them the same amount of care you do someone else you think might become be a regular? It's a big mistake that a lot of practitioners make in all service professions and disciplines including hair salons, spas, restaurants and plenty of other businesses.

> *"We see our customers as invited guests to a party, and we are the hosts. It's our job every day to make every important aspect of the customer experience a little bit better."*
>
> **– Jeff Bezos**

Regardless, I want you to think about what the difference might be if you won that person's business and got them to come back just one more time. At a minimum, if they return for the exact same service and pricing, you're going to at least double your revenue. If they aren't treated very well or they don't get what they need, they'll likely go somewhere else. But if you do a good job in terms of listening and meeting a client's needs, you can win them over from even a small service. And if you can get that person to come back regularly, it can really add up.

A good rule of thumb for many service businesses like massage therapy or energy work, facials, acupuncture, pedicures and some waxing is to get clients to return once a month. Others, such as personal training, chiropractic or physical therapy may be better suited to weekly repetition while still others may be suited for longer periods between visits. For the sake of this example, we'll use the monthly service model as it's become popular over the last decade or so. In fact, if you look many of the franchise models out there, the monthly model is exactly what they honed in on to become successful. As a result, many people now look at a monthly wellness or health service as regular maintenance for themselves just like they would for their car. It's a great rule of thumb to suggest if clients can't afford or budget the time and money more often.

So what happens if you get a new client to come in 12 times a year? In the simplest terms, if your average price is $60, then that translates to $720 coming into your business each year. Not a bad result from simply getting someone new to reschedule once a month! And if you can retain a new client - let's call her Mona - beyond the first year to come for five years, you've added another $2880 to that number. The total so far from getting Mona to come back in and becoming a regular client is $3600. Not bad, right?

Now think about the power of one satisfied, happy, ideal client. When someone is getting great results on their health and wellness goals, and looking or feeling better, those closest to them are bound to notice the difference and ask what they are doing differently. Suddenly, your new ideal monthly client, Mona, has referred two of her friends who both want to do whatever program their friend has.

> **"Make a customer, not a sale."**
>
> **~Katherine Barchetti**

Jennifer, the first person referred by Mona, decides to come in every month for the exact same $60 service she gets and does so for two years, before moving out of the area. The additional income into your business is $1440 dollars.

Hal, he second person referred by Mona (and Jennifer's husband) has a lot of pain issues. He needs more work each session, so he's going to get 90-minute sessions which are $90 each. Like his wife, he comes in once a month and brings another $2160 into your business before he and Jennifer move.

Total income from Mona, Jennifer & Jim over 5 years - $7200

But what about the other things Mona, Jennifer and Hal could spend money on in your business? (Remember, at the beginning of the book I said there were **three** ways to build your business.)One was getting new clients in, one was getting new clients to come back or come in more often, and the third way was to get people to spend more money in your business each visit. This third option can include things like purchasing gift certificates, buying retail or even leaving a great tip. Here are some realistic hypothetical numbers for Mona, Hal and Jennifer to spend over their time with you.

Tips

Mona - $10 per visit x 12 visits per year x 5 years = $600

Jennifer - $10 per visit x 12 visits per year x 2 years = $240

Hal - $20 per visit x 12 visits per year x 2 years = $480

Total Tips - $1,320

Gift Certificates

Mona – 2 x $60 per year (for her sisters) x 5 = $600
Jennifer – 1 x 60 per year (for yoga teacher) x 2 = $120
Hal – 1 x 90 per year (for secretary) x 2 = $180

Total Gift Certificates - $900

So, with those additional sales, we've added another $2220 in revenue for grand total of **$9420** plus at least four new clients

(Mona's sister's, Jennifer's yoga teacher and Hal's secretary – any or all of whom are potential lifetime clients.) This is a HUGE impact...all from treating Mona like a lifetime client and getting her to come back regularly.

Granted, if you are not the business owner, (and even if you are) you will only receive a portion of the total sales, which is totally okay as the business needs to make money so that you continue to have a place to work! Regardless of how it's split, it's important for you to recognize the true impact that taking care of each client every time can make on your business. Take a moment to think about the impact your share of $9520 could have on your life as well.

Next I'm going to give you a real example from my own practice, because I want you to really see the power of following up and taking care of someone.

Doubting Thomas

Thomas started seeing me my first year in practice. After the first visit, he enthusiastically told me the massage felt great and gave me a nice tip! However, when I asked if he wanted to reschedule, he said "no," and walked out the door. For the next few weeks, he came in for massage appointments regularly and we repeated the same scenario several times.

As someone who was trying to build my practice, it really bothered me that he didn't reschedule immediately. I knew he liked my work but wanted to know I could count on him returning, and didn't know what the problem was. Why wouldn't he reschedule?

Finally, after one appointment I asked. "Thomas, I noticed that every time you come in, you enjoy the massage, tell me how great it felt, but then leave without rescheduling. Why is that?"

"Well Felicia, I have many appointments each week and never know my schedule until Monday morning."

Yay! He had an unpredictable schedule and that's why he couldn't rebook. It wasn't me! I thought about his answer for a moment, and said, "Thomas, if I called you on Monday mornings when you know your schedule, would that be helpful to you?"

With a perplexed look on his face, he said, " You'd call me?"

"Sure! I'd be happy to call you on Mondays if that would help you come in for a massage every week."

"Wow, Felicia. That would be great!"

So, guess what I did? It may sound crazy, but for 18 years I called Thomas every single Monday morning to find out if he'd have time for a massage that week. Eventually, we found a standing time which worked well for him, so then I'd call to confirm he could make it.

> The more you engage with customers the clearer things become and the easier it is to determine what you should be doing.
> ~ *John Russell*

Initially, my goal was simply to get Thomas to rebook every week. I wasn't planning for the long-term per se. I was just trying to put a predictable amount of revenue in my pocket each week. However, the special touch of reaching out to him every week made him very loyal.

65

More than twenty one years after his first appointment, Thomas is *still* my client. And although several years ago I started using email to confirm his appointments ahead of time, I still do it. He was, and still is, a real priority to me.

The Impact

Since Thomas travels a lot more for pleasure now than he did when we first started working together, and misses more appointments than he used to, I'd estimate he's averaged about forty massages a year for the last twenty one years, paying an average total of $70 per session including the tip. Let's see how that adds up:

40 Massages a year x $70 a session x 21 years = $63,000

Wow…Thomas has paid me over $60,000 to massage him! Can you believe it?

But that's not all…he also buys gift certificates for his wife, Judy, AKA "The Lifesaver Lady." Judy has been a client as long as Thomas has and comes in about 12 times a year.

12 Massages a year x $70 a session x 21 years = $17,640

Did I mention <u>Judy is one of the best referral sources I've *ever* had</u>? Many of her referrals were (or continue to be) with me for multiple years. The ten clients she's referred to my current practice/spa (open since 2006) have spent a combined **$15,016** on their services so far and have also referred additional clients. And though I no longer have records from my first spa, I can think of at least eight other former regular clients Judy referred – most of whom came in monthly on average for a year or longer – who easily had 175 total sessions between 1994 and 2006. Using the very low end of my prices during that time ($50), these clients would have brought in another **$8750** to my business, though I believe the amount is likely much higher.

Conservatively speaking, here's the cumulative effect of retaining Thomas as a client:

Thomas - 40 massages a year x $70 x 21 years = $63,000

Judy - 12 Massages a year x $70 x 21 years = $17,640

+Income from Judy's Referrals $15,016 + $8750 = $23,766

Total Value of Thomas as a Lifetime Client - $104,406

Do all those Monday morning phone calls still seem crazy to you? Not all clients will be consistently loyal or such avid promoters as Thomas and Judy, but you never know who *your* $104,000 client could be!

SUMMARY

Make it a habit to look at EVERY client as a potential lifetime client, and think of ways you can develop a stronger relationship with them. Often, all it takes to win someone for a lifetime is asking a few questions, making a few phone calls, and remembering to stock up on Lifesavers®.

(Note: For scripts on a variety of rebooking scenarios and tips for making the rebooking process easy check out my book **Free & Easy Ways to Promote Your Massage, Spa & Wellness Business** at www.Spalutins.com and www.EveryTouchMarketing.com)

"In the effort to reach the stars and change the world, make sure you touch a heart and change a life."
— **Stella Payton**

8 BECOME A LIFETIME PROFESSIONAL

If you haven't figured it out by now, it's often the little things, the extras, the unexpected kindnesses as well as the gestures grand and small that touch clients in a meaningful way. In other words, details count along with the big stuff and can be the very thing that win your clients over for a lifetime.

So how do you start to WOW? Begin with WHO!

The most important place to begin is with YOU and doing what is needed to become A FOREVER PROFESSIONAL. What I mean by this is to develop and hone qualities and habits in yourself that make you better or different than anyone else, by being the very best version of yourself with your clients.

I'm not talking about technique training, although it helps greatly to be highly skilled at whatever services you are providing. This of course may take a significant investment on your part in terms of education, products, equipment and practice. But what I'm really talking about is the person you bring to every client encounter and interaction.

So what qualities does a Forever Professional have? Since I own a wellness spa focused on massage therapy, the qualities I'm sharing pertain more specifically to massage therapists - and most have actually been taken directly from reviews and testimonials written about my spa's team. That being said, I think they can apply to anyone who works with clients in a personal service business and go a long way towards building lifetime client relationships.

Qualities and Habits of a Forever Professional
- Thoughtful
- Intuitive
- Professional
- Warm
- Friendly and personable
- Gentle
- Intentional
- Ability to tune in
- Aware
- Welcoming
- Open
- Does a thorough assessment
- Explained process
- Take time to get to know clients
- Provide value added experience
- Knowledgeable
- Attention to detail
- Customized products for me
- Asked what areas to skip
- Checked in about pressure
- Asked questions
- Offered solutions and advice
- Made me comfortable
- Remembered personal details

- Gave a warm greeting
- Attentive
- Respectful
- Good communication
- Puts clients at ease
- Pleasant
- Seamless Flow
- Nurturing
- Pays attention to my needs
- Uses visual aids/pictures
- Provides self care or stretching exercises
- Offers a tour
- Explains services/procedures
- Informative
- Prepared to handle unexpected problems
- Prompt/respectful of clients' time
- Focuses on client's goals
- Stays in touch/checks in between appointments

How many of those qualities or habits do you currently have? Put a check mark by each quality or habit that you are highly adept at now.

Put an X by those you feel are unimportant for you at this time.

Did you see a few that you'd like to add or improve upon? Circle those you want to add or improve and write the top 3 you want to focus on below.

_____

_____

_____

_____

_____

_____

What other qualities or habits would you add to this list?

_____

_____

_____

Now that you've given some thought to WHO you need to be to WOW, let's look at the HOW.

There are TONS of things you can do to set yourself apart and make an indelible impression on your clients that will leave them wanting more. Many resources exist but I will share a few that I have experienced personally in a variety of businesses as well as some things we do in my own office to connect with our valued patrons. Others were things I read about somewhere or which were shared by students/clients over the years but the source is no longer known.

As you read my suggestions and stories, I encourage you to jot down ideas that speak to you or that are sparked by what you're reading. You never know when inspiration will come, so be ready!

Let's start with a few tried and true basics in acknowledging the people who do business with you.

Implement a Welcome or Thank You gift for new clients. As each new client checks in or out for their first visit, thank them for their confidence in choosing your business by giving them a small present or gift bag. If you choose the latter, it can be filled with product samples, coupons for various services, a few referral cards to pass on to friends, or some type of promotional gift with your company's name and contact information on it, such as a pad and pen or coffee mug, etc.

Celebrate your client's birthdays!

If you don't already have a birthday program in place you are losing a great marketing opportunity as well as a lot of revenue. Everyone has a birthday and most people enjoy doing something special to celebrate it.

Make it easy for them to choose your business as a place to celebrate their special day. Send them a postcard or email invitation with a free gift or special offer to help them celebrate their birthday. If your business is small enough for you to write a personal greeting on the card, that is all the better. If not, don't let that stop you. Start by collecting client birthdays in your database or point-of-sale system - and then do something to acknowledge them. Most clients will appreciate the fact you remembered their special day.

Help People Save Time

Partner with a mobile automobile care service that offers wash, wax and details or an oil change at their client's location so that clients can take care of their car while they take care of themselves. You'll probably have to do a little extra work coordinating the details so you may want to work out a referral program or commission split on every car service you arrange. Offer to give the car service coupons or small gift certificates to pass out to their other clients and inform them of the dual offer you have decided to provide. This can work equally well for men and women and will likely introduce a lot of clients to each of your businesses.

Self Care University

Offer fun and interesting classes for your clients. Teach them the basics of proper nail care, special occasion make-up application, massage for hands, neck and shoulders, easy up-dos or braided styles for hair or at home body treatments. Offer first a demonstration and then have each person practice what they have learned on their own or as appropriate, with a partner. Classes can be catered to the time of year…couples massage for Valentine's and during wedding season…makeup lessons prior to the holidays, graduations and wedding season, nail care. Since you are offering instruction as well as a demonstration, you may want to charge a small fee in line with the length of the class. And don't fear that they will learn all your tricks and stop coming in. People will still want to visit the spa for their full relaxation experience, but will appreciate being able to take some of the magic home with them.

Love People's Pet Causes - and Their Pets

Join forces with charities your clients are known to support through their own volunteering and donations - or that have been of help to them when they needed. This type of community involvement can open many new doors for a growing business and help you connect more deeply with clients you already serve.

Support a local or national charity by donating all or a percentage of your sales made on a certain day or date to that cause. You may want to find a well-established cause that has a number of businesses on board already (and is well-known or publicized in your area) or break fresh ground. For example, in 2001 after September 11th, my spa donated 10% of all sales one weekend to the Red Cross.

Years later, we did the same thing again after Hurricane Katrina, both times earmarking our donations for related relief efforts. It will encourage sales that people might otherwise put off or purchases that people would make elsewhere.

One area that can definitely pull on the heart strings strongly is anything to do with pets, especially if your ideal clients are animal lovers. Whether you simply donate a portion of your proceeds for a week or month to a particular organization or you reward clients with a discount for every donation they make, the effort you make to help animals can have a huge feel-good factor.

Stay in Touch with Gratitude

Take time to write old fashioned thank you notes to your clients and vendors, as well as people that you encounter each day. Hand-written thank you notes are really a lost art, so much so that receiving them makes a very big impression. Your note should be warm and genuine as well as professional. Always include a business card and the invitation for them to do business with you in the future.

Nothing says you can only do this with new clients, so take other opportunities to connect with people through the mail, email, social media and even texts. Whatever the message, be sure to remind the recipients how much you appreciate them.

I also include one of my positive thought cards in the notes I send. Many will keep this memento where they can see it even after they toss out the note. Similarly, one past coaching client sends positive encouraging thought or story to her clients each month by email. It is uplifting and beautiful - and her clients love it.

This habit takes time and effort which can be hard to find in a busy life, but you will stand out of the crowd and reap the benefits many times over.

A few other examples:

- My chiropractor chooses a "Patient of the Week" every week.The person is honored with the gift of a plant or flowers and gets their picture taken with the doctor. If the patient chooses, their name and the picture are posted on the office bulletin board behind the check-in desk.

- The garage where I take my car has done a number of fun things over the years to win their clients over. Some of my favorites have included playing big Band or Swing music over their loudspeakers instead of the news or radio. They've also had homemade cookies free at the counter and are happy to give you a ride if needed while your car is being serviced.

- One of my favorite birthday massage experiences was with a past student, Carol, who had a variety of flavored cupcakes waiting for me upon arrival at her office. Before my massage I got to pick the one I wanted and enjoy a sweet treat before my massage. It was very cute, thoughtful and special.

- On a recent birthday, I had a massage session with Aten Doukas, LMBT, a dear friend and past team member from two of my spas. In addition to really feeling like I was being celebrated after a wonderful service, Aten gave me a customized aromatherapy inhaler of oils he knows I like.

Besides my own experiences and suggestions about how to WOW, I asked a few coaching clients and readers to share ideas on how they wow clients. Some of their stories are on the following pages.

Pampering is a Way of Life

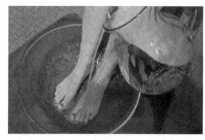

I enjoy pampering my clients from the moment they arrive. Upon arrival, I give my client a warm neck wrap and a foot bath. The neck wrap covers the shoulders and has been warming in the hot towel cabbie. I place a nice fluffy towel on the floor, and on top of the towel I place a

large clear plastic bowl. I ask the client to place their feet in the bowl while I pour warm water infused with lavender body wash over their feet from a pretty clear pitcher. My clients love the extra touch and look forward to the ritual.

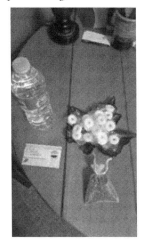

At the end of each appointment the client gets to pick out a self affirmation card out of a basket. I give them the choice of choosing a card by the color or closing their eyes to pick and see what the universe wants them to have. It is amazing that most clients say the card speaks to them that day. Most clients keep the card on their mirror or in the car.

As a gift for my client's first visit I give them a small organza bag filled with pure lavender buds. I mention that they can keep the lavender with them and when they are stressed they can rub the pouch and this releases the oils from the lavender which they can inhale to help de-stress and relax. Some like to do this before they go to sleep and place the bag inside their pillowcase to relax and drift off to sleep.

Anna Carter
Tree of Life Massage & Facial Studio
Rock Hill, SC
www.treeoflifestudio.biz

****

Love My Dog, Love Me

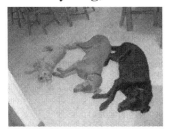

"I do animal massage. I work with athletes, geriatric, injured animals, and hospice. I also do Reiki while I massage.

One thing I do for clients that I haven't heard about other people doing is sending Reiki during troubled times, including death. If one of my clients (I refer to the animal as the client; their person is the owner or parent) is having a crisis that can't be solved by massage, I offer to send distance Reiki at no charge. I let the owner know what time I am sending it, so they can feel comforted by that, as well as (hopefully) the animal.

I also have a complimentary service where, if the animal's time has come, I ask them to tell me the time of euthanasia. At that time, I send Reiki to the pet, owners, and veterinary staff. I worked in a vet clinic for many years and assisted with many euthanasias, and heard many comments about how peaceful it was when I did Reiki. For grieving owners, I will visit them with my dog for a therapy visit. I try not to disappear as soon as my client is gone.

Often when I perform this service, I have lost my client, but the owner is very comforted and doesn't feel abandoned at a very confusing and difficult time. I tend not to think about the business aspect of it, but when that owner does get another animal and that animal needs massage, I am first in their mind. I also get good word of mouth, not to mention good karma.

Lisa Ruthig, Director of Animal Programs
Doggone U at Bancroft School of Massage Therapy
www.HorseAndDogMassage.com
Owner, Lively Dog / Lively Horse Massage Therapy & Reiki
www.LivelyDog.net

****

Chocolate IS Healing

I work in Connecticut where it can get really COLD. In the winter months, when people are tired and sun deprived, I share with them my other

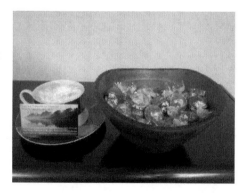

passion besides massage, **chocolate.** And not the cheap stuff! I delight them with a rich cup of hot chocolate before or after their massage, and they also get a wickedly delicious gourmet chocolate truffle for the ride home. They don't forget this magic combination and they keep coming back for more.

Peter A Heimuller, L.M.T.
Owner - Cloud 9 Therapeutic Massage
Danbury, CT
Cloud 9 Therapeutic Massage

****

Every Season is Special

My special touches are seasonal. During the cooler months I treat my clients to a warm cup of homemade cocoa or apple cider to help warm up their bodies before or after a massage. The summer months I have tester bottles of sun screen to apply before heading out in the evening sun. And every new client gets a goodies bag of samples from Bon Vital that I use for any and all my services with a special discount if they rebook within 60 days.

DeAnn Holexa
Boise, ID
www.deann.massagetherapy.com

****

What special touches have you been wowed by?

_____

_____

_____

_____

_____

And finally...Lydia Smith, a massage industry veteran from Florida shared two wonderful examples of wowing both prospective and long-term clients.

#1 Creating Value

I give my clients, most who've been coming to see me for twenty years or longer, free organic produce from my vegetable garden in Florida. When I travel to Michigan, I get them organic hand-picked (by me) apples of various varieties as well as various homegrown squashes and potatoes from the garden of friends in Michigan. My 24+ year clients also get home-raised honey from the private Michigan beehives and organic blueberries.

#2 Everyone Knows Someone

In 1988 when I was first starting, I handed out business cards to everyone. One day, at my part time job at the Ice Cream Churn, a lady came in upset. Her car was overheating.

I went out with her to fix her radiator – adding water to the dry radiator. We talked about life, stress and I handed her my card. Two months later she came in, loved my work and referred all her jazz musician clients to me. She was my client for 5 years and the total monetary return (from meeting her) was roughly $51,000 due to all the great professional international musicians I met.

Lydia Smith
Beneficial Massage
Mt. Dora, FL

Here are a few suggestions for other special touches YOU can add to make any personal service or appointment feel more special.

- Keep fresh flowers in your office or waiting area (including on a treatment table)
- Provide complimentary grooming or dental hygenie products in your bathrooms. This could include hand lotion, hair spray, mouth wash, and so on.
- Have feminine products accessible without having to ask
- Keep hard candies and emergency cough drops close by
- Be prepared for wardrobe emergencies with a supply of safety pins and or a sewing kit
- Have a complimentary beverage station with herbal tea, coffee, water and other drinks
- Have light snacks available for clients who are in a rush (granola bars, fresh fruit, etc)
- Keep umbrellas by your front door for clients to borrow in the rain - or offer to walk them to their cars in a storm
- Offer free wi-fi or electronic device charging. Bonus points if you keep an array of chargers available
- Send holiday cards
- Follow up with clients when you haven't heard from them in a while, just to say hello or check to see how they are doing.
- If you use products, send clients home with a sample of what you used with them during the appointment
- Listen - really listen - to what they are saying

What are some other special touches you can add to win your clients over for a lifetime?

_____

_____

_____

SUMMARY

In short, there are countless ways to make people feel special, but the ones that work best are the ones you actually do - and that come from your heart. Take time to brainstorm about how you want to connect with your clients in a special way and then take action on putting those ideas into place.

9 FIRING NON-IDEAL CLIENTS

So far I've talked a lot about ideal, lifetime clients as well as how to find them. One thing I haven't yet mentioned is non-ideal clients and how to let them go. That's our next step.

But first let's talk about exactly what a bad client is. If you've been in business long, you probably already know who I'm talking about, and may even be picturing one or two of yours in your mind's eye as you read this. These folks aren't necessarily bad people - although they could be - but tend to exhibit one or more less-than-charming or "bad" behaviors.

Non-ideal clients may...

- Habitually show up late, unhelpfully early, stay too long, or a combination of the three.
- Often come in rushed, stressed, or in a bad mood, putting you into a negative state of mind.
- Be overly demanding, needy, hard to please and/or an incessant complainer
- Have personal hygiene issues
- Expect ongoing discounts or deals because they are such loyal customers, yet brag about how much money they make, have or spent somewhere else

83

- Give unsolicited advice because they know more than you do – about everything
- Expect more energy and time from you than the service allows - or than they are willing to pay for
- Cancel or change their appointments at the last minute or "no-show" without calling
- Be loud, nosy, negative, rude, arrogant, disrespectful or snobby
- Have no regard for the personal space or boundaries of others
- Act inappropriately or be socially inept
- Want you to do things out of your area of expertise or scope of practice
- Fail to pay promptly
- Wear you out, bring you down or get on your last nerve
- And the list goes on

Besides this laundry list of potential faults and faux pas, some non-ideal clients are simply a bad fit for you.

Another Man's Treasure

When I was first in practice, I worked for Joel Tull ,the owner of The Human Touch, then a group massage practice. One week, when Joel was away to run in a marathon out of state, I saw several of his regular clients. Though I was very grateful for the extra income, it was immediately apparent that his ideal clients were not mine.

One of these folks was a young woman whom I'll call Michelle. Michelle was a runner, probably about thirty five years old, and had a terse, tense disposition. With most of my regulars, each appointment started off with some friendly banter, Michelle stomped in with a frown on her face and did not want to talk to me. Instead she sighed heavily as we began the session, clearly displeased to be seeing me instead of her usual therapist. I asked Michelle a few questions initially to try and break the ice, but quickly realized she was not interested in sharing anything beyond her requirements for the session.

As the massage progressed, I uncovered her feet and found she still had her socks on. Surprised I asked, "Are your feet ticklish or something?"

"No. I always leave them on. Joel takes them off for me and then puts them back on after he rubs my feet."

Now, as a more seasoned practitioner, it wouldn't bother me at all to do this for one of my clients, whether they were a regular or first timer. However, at that point in my career, and perhaps because Michelle and I had no connection or rapport between us, I felt her expectation was very demanding and didn't want to do it. I also immediately knew she was not an ideal client for me, and happily turned her back over to her regular sock-removing practitioner.

"I strongly recommend breaking up with any client who zaps your energy. They will take away from the good things that you have to offer the next client on your book. If you constantly surround yourself with clients who make you feel good you WILL get more referrals, retail sales and your up-selling skills will improve....Remember- countless studies have shown that being around positive people will reduce stress and improve your immune system. This is a must to ensure high performance on your part as a successful practitioner."

Lori Crete
Author of **The Six Figure Esthetician System**

Identifying the Bad Guys

So how do you get rid of undesirable customers and replace them with ideal clients? Start by knowing the difference between who you want and who you don't. If you still aren't sure who your ideal client is, go back to **Chapter 3 (Your Ideal Lifetime Clients)** and re-read it as well as your own ideal client description(s).

"If it was necessary to tolerate in other people everything that one permits oneself, life would be unbearable."

~ Georges Courteline

While my list of non-ideal behaviors and story above illustrate many potential issues you could encounter, it is not necessarily an accurate picture of issues you find undesirable in your clients. With the next exercise, you should be able to identify the folks that do not fit the picture or description of your ideal clients. Before you set off "firing" anyone in your business, take a moment to determine exactly which negative qualities, actions or behaviors you want to eliminate or avoid in your own clientele.

Deal Breaker Exercise

Circle each client issue you find difficult to deal with.

- Habitually show up late, unhelpfully early, stay too long, or a combination of the three.
- Often come in rushed, stressed, or in a bad mood, putting you into a negative state of mind.
- Be overly demanding, needy, hard to please and/or an incessant complainer
- Have personal hygiene issues

- Expect ongoing discounts or deals because they are such loyal customers, yet brag about how much money they make, have or spent somewhere else
- Give unsolicited advice because they know more than you do – about everything
- Expect more energy and time from you than the service allows - or than they are willing to pay for
- Cancel or change their appointments at the last minute or "no-show" without calling
- Be loud, nosy, negative, rude, arrogant, disrespectful or snobby
- Have no regard for the personal space or boundaries of others
- Act inappropriately or be socially inept
- Want you to do things out of your area of expertise or scope of practice
- Fail to pay promptly
- Wear you out, bring you down or get on your last nerve

What other qualities, actions or behaviors do you consider to be less than ideal?

_____

_____

_____

_____

From the lists above of qualities, habits or activities, which issues are absolute deal breakers with your clients?

_____

_____

_____

Bad Clients/Non-Ideal Clients

Jot down the names of a few people who are either not your ideal clients and whom you need to let go of, or who may need to be rehabilitated from their bad behavior. Next to their name write down the reason why they need to go. If you think they can be rehabilitated, put a check by their name. If not, begin thinking about your break-up plan as you read the next section.

_____

_____

_____

_____

_____

_____

"When breaking up with a client...own it. Don't make it their fault. If you say, "You need to find another therapist because of your actions," they can counter with, "I will be better." I tell them that I am no longer the therapist for you, but I shall help you find the right therapist for you.

_If they ask what they did, I say, "It's not you. It is me and my decision." If they press, I say, "I feel that I cannot do my best work here and you deserve only the best. I know a therapist that I think would work for you. His name is _____ and here is his number."_

Susie Byrd
Director & Instructor
The Edge School of Massage
Fayetteville, Arkansas

Let Them See Themselves Out

Before you start lining up people for the chopping block, I want you to consider making a few changes that will allow non-ideal clients to determine for themselves whether they should stay or move on.

1. **Focus on doing what you love and eliminate the services you don't enjoy.** If you aren't clear on this, go back to **Chapter 4 (Doing What You Love for a Lifetime)** and re-read the section on Passion as well as your answers for the exercise that followed. Sometimes the reason we think of someone as an undesirable client has nothing to do with them and everything to do with what we've been doing with them.

   In my own practice, I found this to be true with a pain relief modality I used to offer. Though I've found it to be very effective with some people, and seemingly easier than doing a massage, it totally drains me every time I do it. This is unfortunate since it is less time-consuming than my usual appointments. However, I dreaded doing it and found myself exhausted after every fifteen to twenty minute session. Thus, I took it off my website and stopped inviting my massage clients to try it. Eventually, I hope someone else in my spa will have a desire to learn it and I can refer people to them.

2. **Set, communicate and enforce clear boundaries and policies with your clients.** It is possible some "bad" clients developed negative habits because they didn't know your policies or rules. In effect, you gave them permission to behave badly by not defining or explaining your expectations of them initially or after the first infraction occurred. (This is quite common in service-based and helping professions.)

   Professional policies typically cover things like no-shows and cancellations, late-arrivals, and illness/emergency situations, but may also discuss how you handle discounts, payments, children, confidentiality, etc.) You should feel good enough about each policy to easily explain and comfortably enforce them. Once you are happy with the policies communicate these with all clients – and enforce them with smiling regularity. Though it may seem easier to let folks be exempt from the rules or make exceptions because you don't want to upset someone in the moment, this can cause bigger problems or headaches for everyone in the long term.

And while some rule-breakers are simply unknowingly being inconsiderate, others will unknowingly take advantage of your seemingly accommodating manner, not realizing that they are acting badly by exhibiting whatever negative behavior they've turned into a chronic and potentially damaging habit.

3. **Modify your schedule.** In my own practice, I've found many clients who are challenging for me to work with like to come in on the days and times I least like to work. Perhaps this is because I'm not adequately rested or would rather be doing something fun instead of being at work. Over time, I've learned what hours and days work best for me as well as recognizing when I need to take time for myself. You should consider adjusting your schedule in ways which will allow you and your clients to have the best experiences and outcomes possible.

4. **Increase your prices.** One way to drop a few non-ideal clients from your schedule is to raise your prices. This is usually the bargain shoppers or those who've been complaining about your fees. Charging higher prices will also attract new clients who value your time and services more –

90

and allow you to make more money. If you're concerned you'll lose some of your favorite people because they can't afford the increase, know that you can choose to make an exception here and there, or to create a program or package that will keep them at the old rate.

For ideas on packages I've used with tremendous success, check out my book, **Free & Easy Ways to Promote Your Massage, Spa & Wellness Business** *at EveryTouchMarketing.com*

Though increasing your prices may not be an option if you work in someone else's business, it's always worth a conversation with your boss. Explain your perspective and reasoning - you may be surprised at the outcome.

> "We are constantly being put to the test by trying circumstances and difficult people and problems not necessarily of our own making."
>
> ~ Terry Brooks

5. **Client Rehab**. Sometimes you can effectively address the conflict as a first (or final) step before firing them. In the conversation you want to identify the problem or conflict, explain why this is a problem, and identify what specific changes or steps you want to see happen.

Here's a sample conversation with a client who's habitually late.

"Seth, I really love working with you and want to continue to do so until we can get rid of your old acne scars. However, it's really important we

91

start our sessions on time. When we don't, I run late the rest of the day and feel very stressed out. Will you help me feel less stress by arriving ten minutes before your appointment time so we can stay on schedule?"

When your client feels appreciated and understands exactly what you want or need from them to improve the situation, you're more likely to get the results you want and transform that person into an ideal client. If such a conversation doesn't work, then it can actually pave the way to sending them on to someone else, or not seeing them anymore.

Walk Them to the Door

Address the mismatch directly. Despite your best efforts to change or improve some client behaviors and habits, some people will not get the message or adhere to the new policies you've set. Though many clients will fire themselves by choosing not to adapt to a new schedule or pricing, the ones who don't will be left for you to deal with. In cases that cannot be improved or rehabbed, it will be time to let the clients go. Firing a client isn't necessarily easy, but that doesn't mean it's not necessary. And though this type of situation can be difficult or painful, professional break-ups can often be handled with grace, and compassion.

If possible, refer them to another professional or business. Long ago, I learned to have a variety of referral sources for people in the same and similar businesses for this very reason. If you know someone who would be a better fit for a client, who can actually help them with the problem or goal they have, (or works the hours they want to come in, charges a lower price, is in their neighborhood, etc.) then be willing to give a referral to the non-ideal client.

This is one of the reasons why I strongly encourage all personal service professionals to network with their colleagues and get to know each other, or to trade/purchase services from each other. When you've actually experienced other people's work, you're able to give them referrals with confidence. Except for the worst of the worst, chances are that our "bad clients" are in fact, someone else's ideal customers. With a little research and relationship development, you can develop a good network of referral resources within your area or community, and often within your own company if you have multiple people who do related work.

Hate doing pre-natal massage? Find someone who adores working with expectant moms and ask them to send you all the stressed out dads. Detest doing "pampering-only" skin care or bodywork services? Send your relaxation clients to one who truly adores blending aromatherapy with ambiance instead of providing medically-based or results-driven treatments. Also look to align yourself with other professionals who work opposing hours or in different neighborhoods to provide an assortment of options for clients that are not your best fit.

Here's my story about referring a non-ideal client to someone else…

Shirley's Sick

My first solo office was in a personal training gym. Because of its small size and personalized nature, there were quite a few members I got to know pretty well before they became my clients. One of them, Shirley, a dental assistant for over thirty years and had trained at the gym for quite a while. As with many members, I'd see Shirley at the gym several times a week as well as socially on a few occasions. We often chatted while she was on the treadmill, which I really enjoyed.

Since we'd met a few months earlier, Shirley had been to me for massage a couple times, and both appointments had gone well. However perhaps because we had that casual relationship, she felt more comfortable with me than she would have otherwise, which may be what caused the following situation to occur the way it did.

Shirley had an appointment with me at 9 AM on a Tuesday morning, my first appointment of the day. When she arrived for her session, I was sitting at my desk with my back to the door. I turned around as I heard her walk in and was shocked to see her laboring into the room wearing a nightgown. As she dragged herself closer to where I sat, I nervously asked, "Oh my gosh, Shirley, what's wrong?"

Breathlessly she said "I've been SO sick," and continued to tell me about the illness she'd had over the last few days. Her whole body was weak, aching and tired. Red flag.

"Shirley, have you had a fever?" I questioned.

"Oh yeah."

Houston we have a problem. I can't do a massage on someone with a fever. "Have you had the fever in the last 24 hours?"

"Yes, until last night," she said with a panic in her eye.

So I calmly said to her "Shirley, you know, it's a contraindication to massage someone who's had a fever in the last 24 hours. I think we better reschedule."

Shirley paused for a moment before saying anything. "Oh, but I thought the massage would make me feel so much better, and I've been looking forward to this *all weekend*. I just (holding back tears)… I **really** want to feel better. Can't you do it?!"

What happened next was really shocking. As Shirley's emotion-filled words poured from her lips, I felt an all too familiar wave of guilt rise up and over me. Paralyzed and wanting to stop the flow of guilt from drowning me, I stammered, "Okay, okay, okay. I'll do the massage," steeling myself after the unexpected turn of events.

Let me explain.

Shirley's reaction was an unknowingly spot-on rendition of a very classic behavior - a guilt trip - of my mother's, particularly when she didn't get what she wanted, and especially if she was sick, which was often. (Sorry, Mom!) In an instant, Shirley turned into my mom in front of my very eyes and I caved as a way to stop the emotional roller coaster in it's tracks . What happened to me was an immediate transformation back into a teenage girl who didn't know how to deal with manipulation from her mother or anyone else. In the massage world, we know this as transference and counter-transference.

After that I, basically stepped over my own boundaries and policies to let Shirley into my world, and as a result she kind of sucked me dry. As I worked on her, I began to feel weak, tired and totally drained of energy. My body started feeling achy and feverish, and my throat started hurting. I felt so terrible, in fact, that within minutes of starting the appointment, I started making a list in my head of who I needed to call when we finished – my doctor and all the clients I was going to cancel for the day.

When the session was over, I felt like death warmed over. By contrast, Shirley practically bounced off the table and said "Wow, I feel great!" before skipping out the door. I collapsed on the couch in my waiting room before rescheduling all of my clients for the day.

Once I had a chance to think about what happened, I knew I needed to fire Shirley. Now you might be thinking my decision to fire a client based on one isolated incident was a bit rash. It was just one appointment, one conversation, and one sick day. What's the big deal?

I had to fire Shirley because I reacted to her the way I would have with my mother, which was not good. In fact, it was a very unbalanced response from me – both of us really. Though it might not be immediate, I realized it would only be a matter of time before Shirley would invade my boundaries again and I'd likely respond in the same unhealthy way. Despite liking her as a person and having no other incidents or issues, I knew I couldn't see her as a client again.

Here's the basic conversation we had the next time Shirley called to schedule an appointment.

"Shirley, I'm terribly sorry but I can't schedule you for a massage. I really don't know how to say this, but the truth is you remind me a lot of my mother. She died a few years ago and, unfortunately, we didn't get along that well. When I saw you last time after you'd been sick, some old issues came up for me which have been difficult to deal with. I just can't continue seeing you as a client as a result."

After explaining why I could not see her again, I referred Shirley to a therapist who worked with me and who I thought would be a good fit for her.

It wasn't easy, and mind you, Shirley didn't like hearing what I had to say. She didn't want to see another practitioner, and tried pretty hard to convince me - with another guilt trip - to change my mind. However, I stood my ground and she went to the other therapist. I hope she eventually understood.

Don't Let the Door Hit You

Don't feel obligated to refer your non-ideal clients to anyone. In fact, there are some people you aren't going to refer at all. Referring someone you don't want because they've harmed or mistreated you in some way is a big no-no. This can totally back-fire, creating ill will or negative feelings between you and your colleagues.

When you cannot refer someone to another business - whether due to a lack of options or because their behavior would not allow you to do so with a clear conscience - you may be forced to simply terminate your professional relationship. This is typically not a time to be angry or condemning, but one where you'll want to provide specific reasons or evidence explaining why you are terminating the relationship. A few suggestions:

- Practice what you plan to say so when the time comes, you are prepared to have the discussion in a calm, compassionate manner.
- Write an outline or notes with the key points so you don't forget anything.
- Begin by expressing gratitude for the person's past business.
- Explain why you no longer feel you can service their needs (ex: past difficulties with keeping appointments, etc.)
- Have the proof to back you up if needed, but leave out the blame and finger pointing.
- Hold your ground. If you've thought this through and made a decision to let someone go, honor your choice.

Here's what the conversation might sound like:

"Bob, I want to thank you for your past business and support of me as a personal trainer. I greatly appreciate it. Unfortunately, due to our ongoing scheduling difficulties, I think it would be best for us to end our professional relationship for the time being. I don't think I can meet your scheduling needs and hope you understand."

SUMMARY
Ending professional relationship can be tough no matter what the circumstances are. However, by letting go of non-ideal clients, you'll be happier and healthier while bringing your business to a higher level of profitability, performance and quality.

"Use your senses to SEE yourself for who you truly are. SMELL the flowers and become one with nature. TASTE the goodness of God. HEAR the truth. TOUCH the hearts of others with kindness and honest deeds."
— **Amaka Imani Nkosazana**
in **Heart Crush**

10 CONCLUSION

Regardless of the profession you're in, the products or services you provide, or even whether you own the business or simply work in it, finding and keeping the clients who are a perfect fit for you today, tomorrow and for a lifetime is the key to creating a career that is enjoyable, rewarding and prosperous.

Though I've outlined what I feel are my best suggestions for reaching and retaining customers who are ideal for you and your company, they are just a start. Use the suggestions I've made to spark your own creativity along with an ongoing discovery process about what makes your patrons tick, spend, refer and return. Talk to them often about their needs, wants, likes, dislikes, problems and preferences. Keep the lines of communication open both ways and encourage their feedback often.

Also, look at what other companies are doing to woo, win, and wow their clientele, even if they are in a totally different industry. There are many great examples to learn from and emulate. You may also want to find out what your competition is doing well through reading reviews or paying a personal visit to them.

Likewise, continue to stay in touch with yourself about what you need, like and want out of your business and clients. Like your clients, your preferences and desires may change from time to time. What you are passionate about today may evolve and change as may your field, area and clients.

Being in business for yourself – whether on your own, as a part of a larger enterprise, or at the head of a growing company can be exciting, life enriching and profitable, though not always at the same time! However, despite the inevitable surprises and bumps along the road, if you can keep your focus on doing what you love with people you love working with, the ride will feel much smoother!

YOU ARE A PROFESSIONAL!
YOU DESERVE SUCCESS!
YOU CAN DO THIS!

If you feel so inclined, I'd LOVE to hear how you are creating amazing experiences for your own lifetime clients. Please feel free to email them to me at Felicia@Spalutions.com for possible inclusion in a future book or blog.

Thank you for your time, attention and interest in what I have to say. If you've found this book helpful, please share it with others who might enjoy it, post a review on Amazon, or drop me a note to tell me what you liked best☺ You can also connect with me online☺

Facebook - /FeliciaBrownLMBT and Facebook Page - Spalutions
LinkedIn - /feliciaebrown
Twitter @FeliciaBrown
MassageMag Blog
www.massagemag.com/massage-blog/marketing-with-every-touch/

11 CAREER OF A LIFETIME
AN INTERVIEW WITH BENNY VAUGHN
A SPORTS MASSAGE LEGEND

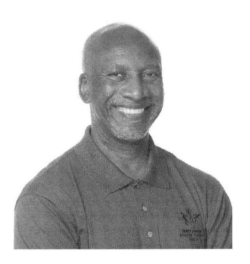

Benny Vaughn, a four time Olympic massage therapist, has set a standard in the United States for Orthopedic Sports Massage Therapy for over four decades. MASSAGE Magazine named him one of the most influential massage therapists in the last 100 years for his contributions in both education and clinical applications of soft-tissue therapy and bodywork. **Benny Vaughn brings over 40 years of focused expertise in soft-tissue manual therapy to his teaching.**

For as long as I've been a massage therapist, I've heard about Benny Vaughn. Though at first I didn't know who he was, it quickly became evident that he was someone highly revered and knowledgeable. Yet, our paths did not cross until a few years ago when I met him in Atlanta. Though the conversation was brief, he was quite cordial and respectful to me as a fellow educator.

Then a year or two later, I had a chance to interview him one-on-one for use in a future book. Although I wasn't quite sure what to expect to hear in an interview focused on business since he is best known for his Sports Massage expertise, I quickly discovered that Benny has been quite masterful and deliberate in creating his own thriving practice.

Even if you are not a massage therapist, this interview sheds light on why Benny has been successful as a business owner and massage professional. I hope it will give you some ideas about how to create a highly successful career, whatever your field.

****

This is Felicia Brown. I'm here talking with Benny Vaughn. Bennie would you do me a favor as we're getting started and just tell me a little about your credentials, what you're known for and so on?

Okay, my name is Benny Vaughn. That's spelled B-e-n-n-y V-a-u-g-h-n. I have been a massage therapist since 1976. I'm a practicing massage therapist and what I mean by that is I still go to work each day and do massage. That's how I make my living.

How many clients do you see a day or a week?

An average day I see seven clients a day, sometimes upwards to ten.

Wow.

And I do that five days a week. So you can do the math, 35 to 45 sessions a week is what I do.

Are they all massage or is some of that personal training or athletic training?

It's all massage.

Wow!

Now, I incorporate my knowledge and skill set from athletic training into massage in terms of orthopedic assessment, sometimes advising a client on steps they should take to resolve the issue particularly if they need to be referred to other healthcare providers, such as chiropractic, medical doctor, osteopathic care, acupuncturists and so on.

Fantastic. So, you said you've been in practice for almost 40 years. What's the secret for your longevity and success in the business?

There are areas that I found make a difference in longevity and the first area is take care of yourself physically and mentally. That means train for massage in the same way that an athlete trains for a sporting event. You should do exercise, that includes both strength training, using some of resistance or weighs or body weight and you should do endurance training, cardio vascular training, walking, running, cycling, swimming; any type of activity that helps you to sustain endurance.

So, the first secret that I use is to take care of yourself in the same fashion that an athlete takes care of herself to prepare for an athletic event. Number two, and I should add flexibility, make sure you're stretching too. So strength training, cardio-vascular training, and flexibility, those are things that allow you too physically and mentally and mentally do good massage because you're not hurting, you're not in pain.

The second secret to my success in my massage practice is making each massage session a good experience for the client. It has to be a good experience and it has to be a good experience on every level. What they see, what they hear, what they smell, and what they feel. And what I mean by that what does your massage area look like? What do they see when they come into that area? Are the colors soothing? Do they see pictures or paintings? Do they see sunlight? Do they see things that make them feel good? Do they smell things that make them feel good?

I'm of the neutral approach because we don't always know what each client will respond to, but there are times where you might use an essential oil and a diffusor to create an aroma in the area that is conducive to a good therapeutic experience. But I pick and choose those very, very carefully. I avoid heavily scented candles and heavily scented oils, this sort of thing. But I do use eucalyptus, lavender, menthols, peppermints, occasionally. So, what the person smells and a good office is one where they smell very little so they feel neutral, in my view.

The third piece to success of the experience is what they hear. Have music that engages the client, that helps the client to feel relaxed and welcome, and it doesn't always have to be a low tone music, but I play a wide variety of what I call world music and music in my office comes in seven different languages and I pick and choose based on the time of day and the client that's coming in.

If I know that there's a client who especially likes Reggae, than Reggae music is playing when they arrive. If I have a client that especially likes Blues than Blues is playing when they arrive. And then there are others who just simple like any kind of music that's different than what they are accustom too. In Texas where I am, during rodeo session, I play Country Western music and people appreciate that. We get them in the mood. On St. Patrick's Day we play Celtic music in the office. During the holidays we play all variety of holiday music in five different languages, so what they hear.

What they feel, the texture of the sheets, the texture of your towels, the texture of the table, the texture of the chair that they sit in to take their shoes off, the texture of your office, because we're about sensory experience with people and that sensory experience translates into a good session for that client all the way around. So, it's really important to pay close attention to your actual setup. You want your massage setup to be one that you enjoy being in and working in and that you love being in your massage area; so, putting time into that.

One of the things I have in my, the reception area when a person arrives is I have no right angle edges on desk or tables when they enter. Everything is either round or rounded edges because it invites people to approach the desk for the intake and history that I do with them. It helps people to feel comfortable. Now that could be some sort of Feng Shui thing; I'm not formally trained in any of it, but what I do know is what I see and what makes people feel comfortable.

So, here's some things that I've done in my work area that I believe contributes to the success of a great massage experience. Number #1: The entrance; and remember long before the person ever gets onto the treatment table the massage session has already begun.

And it really begins when you speak to them on the telephone. So, phrases that you use on the telephone with that client when you're booking that appointment with them already begins the massage session. I use phrases like 'I'm looking forward to working with you.' I use phrases such as 'I can help you.' I use phrases such as 'I've seen this before and we can work with this.' I use phrases that give people hope before they even arrive, so the session's already begun.

Now the person arrives. The door to your practice, whether you're in a building that you rent space or some freestanding building, I like to have the first door that the client arrives at a door that the client can see through and see into the area that they're coming. Now sometimes that requires you having to put in a new door. Sometimes those doors are already there. So, it can be a glass door that comes into the building that then leads to your office.

So, let's say you're in an office building; so they have glass doors that come into the main lobby, they look on the directory, they see you're in Suite 210, so they go to Suite 210. So, now they have another door they have to enter. Solid doors are not inviting, especially for massage. So, with the landlord's permission have a vision panel put in the door so people can see in to where they're going. It reduces apprehension. So, that makes a big difference when people feel like, especially for massage, wow this is where I'm going. And then you can also showcase the beauty of your office.

Number #2: put a 'welcome' mat at the front of your door so it can be a saffron color, something that's very soothing and welcoming. I use a saffron color and I have just a mat at the front door of my office and I have a vision panel in the door so people can actually see into the office. Now, they can't see into the actual massage space but the office where I have my desk for the intake history and all, so we have a saffron color welcome mat, we have a vision panel they can see inside the office, they feel welcomed.

All the edges of the tables as they approach are all rounded so that it invites them to come in and be comfortable. In the waiting area, and I don't call it a waiting area because a big part of my success in massage is that I start on time. Start on time. Now, on the surface that doesn't sound like much, but think of all the services we go to that never start on time, so why do I have a reservation at this time with my doctor when I'm forced to sit in the waiting area. Remember the waiting area is a medical doctor creation, the waiting area. We don't need a waiting area.

I have an area that I call the reading area. I have a reading area so when a person comes, they arrive early; make yourself comfortable in the reading area. And in the reading area it's essential that you have current reading material. If you're going to have periodicals, journals, magazines, have something that's at least within the last two months and nothing that was two years ago that we so often see in medical offices. Even my doctor I go to, in the exam room there's a Time magazine from seven years ago. I won't even touch it. I mean how many sick people have touched that magazine? Think about it.

So, have current reading material because when you pay attention to details like that it makes you successful because your clients pay attention to that. They notice that you care enough to pay attention to current reading material. So, I have a reading area, not a waiting area. Because as soon as you tell people, well you can just wait there in the waiting area, they're already beginning to get the idea of 'oh I have to wait. I thought my appointment was at 1 it was at 2.' So, I call it the reading area and you make the reading area comfortable because sometimes a friend may come with your appointment and they need a comfortable place to read and rest while their person receives a massage.

In the treatment room success of the session, or creating a good experience, I use a sound oasis machine in the office. Typically it's tuned into waves breaking on the beach, but some sort of sound oasis that's turned down low where you have this nice ambient sound that's soothing. I have appropriate music playing throughout the office and the treatment tables are heated.

I use a heating pad underneath the sheepskin, the faux sheepskin pad, and then I have the cover table sheet, etc. So, even in the summertime when you think well gosh isn't it warm enough, when you're lying still on a table in an air conditioned room people still get chilly. So, it's easier to cool a person than to try to warm them up. So pay close attention to the temperature comfort of the client and cover them appropriately. So, I have heated tables; they are covered with nice feeling flannel sheet, make sure your sheets feel good to touch and we have all types of sheets available to the massage profession.

And then have the appropriate blankets. The cover that I like a lot are the quilt forters that are made by a company on the Internet whose name I can't remember right now. But they make a great sheet and things. They're handmade in the USA so they're not coming from Pakistan or somewhere where apparently they don't use the same measuring tools as we do because I've worn those sheets before and none of them have right angles and none of them are the same size and they're made in Pakistan – sorry. I'm being ethnocentric or whatever. I'm just telling the truth. The sheets that are made there are crappy. Period.

These sheets are made up in Maine somewhere, New Hampshire, by Americans in a community. They're hand sewn and they do great work and I apologize, I can't remember the name of them but I can send it to you. But they make a blanket called a quiltforter. So, it's like a comforter and a quilt combined, much lighter and it just feels good and it's made out of organic cotton and unfortunately the last time I spoke with them they told me there were looking to discontinue those because they're pretty labor intensive. But I'm hoping they've changed their minds because so many massage therapists like me keep calling and asking for them to come back again. But find some sort of blanket that's comfortable that helps people stay warm and feels good.

Feel free to take a sip of water, or a breath whenever you need to!:-)

So those are things that make a difference. Now let's talk about how do I earn money with massage? How do I make that steady? I do real well annually when I file my taxes. I mean it supports myself and my family. We have a home, we have cars, and I do all of this with massage. So your fee structure is the first point. And you have to decide what you want to charge and it's really up to you what you want to charge.

Now, some would say well you have to see what the market will bear and this and that and all these formulas and what's the massage therapist in the other county charging? None of that really matters in reality. That stuff is MBA theoretical stuff that grad students getting an MBA have to do to justify the MBA. It might work in manufacturing, it might work in building construction, it does not work in massage. You charge what you feel like you want to charge and the people who feel like they want to pay that will come to you. It's really that simple folks.

Yes, you're not going to be able to massage everyone and you can't anyway because you don't have enough time in the day or the strength or willingness to do it. But you have to decide how can I make a comfortable living that will pay my lease, pay the mortgage on my home, although me to travel, do the other things I need to do, pay for healthcare, insurance, or whatever it is you need, and you just simply work from there. So, I decided on – well let me just put it this way, when I began my massage in 1974, I was getting $3.00 a massage for a 30 minute massage.

Wow.

And I got $7.50 a massage for an hour massage; that's $7.50 and I got $3.00 for a 30-minute massage, okay. That's what I got paid and I thought I was big time. I don't remember minimum wage was in 1974 but I think this was a little better than minimum wage and it was interesting work for me. So, I worked at a health club and that's what I got paid. And I'd see, I'd do like 12-14 30-

minute massages. It was factory work but I got a lot of hours in, a lot of experience. So, if I did 14 half-hour massages in the course of a day, I made…what's that $42.00?

I'm definitely not the math girl. $42.00.

Yeah, and I was happy to get that. And so I went from getting a high of $7.50 and then I progressed up; I got $10.00 for an hour of massage work, and now I'm up to a first visit of $180.00, and then single therapy sessions are $130.00. And then the way that you can drive your financial success is sell prepaid accounts and I call them accounts. I used to call them packages, so either one works well but I like the term account. So, I offer clients prepaid accounts and what that means is they pay upfront, they pay in advance in order to get a reduced rate on the per visit fee.

How much would you say you reduce that just on an average? Let's say someone signs up for 20, how much of a reduction is that would you guess?

This is how I do it. So a single session is $130.00, the best account that I offer people, I call it my Platinum account and its $880.00 for eight sessions so that's a $110.00 a session. So, they are saving $160.00.

Gotcha.

By doing that. So, from $130.00 for a single session to $110.00 per session so they save $160.00 over time by buying the Platinum account. Then I have a Gold account where it's six sessions at $115.00 a session and then I have a Silver account where they get four sessions at $120.00. So, depending on what they want to invest in and sometimes I will tell the person, well this particular challenge that you have I'm confident that in four sessions we can have this moving in the right direction for you. And I suggest to them you might want to purchase the Silver account.

You were talking about the names of kind of a way, the Platinum, Gold, Silver, as a way to give people an impression about it. You know it makes them feel good about it. Tell me the other marketing tool that you've used with those kinds of accounts. Something that helped create an impression, make people feel special.

Words make a big difference for people. When you travel on the airlines everybody wants to be Platinum, Executive Platinum, VIP lounge, the Admirals Lounge, the King's Lounge, all these sorts of things. People deserve to feel important because they are important. So, I use the terms Platinum, Gold, and Silver. Sometimes you can use VIP account, but one of the other ways that I've used is to use a Signature Card.

So, you have a Signature Card printed and it just says, has a place where you put the person's name, perhaps their address, their contact number and then you have 10, 15, 20 lines where they can sign on a card and that card should be printed on good, nice, expensive feeling cardstock. It's got to feel important to them and a person can prepay for say you offer them after the Platinum, which is eight in my system, let's say you come up with Executive Platinum or Executive Platinum VIP, 20 sessions, now they're getting 20 sessions at $100.00 a session. So, they pay you $2,000 in advance for that.

So, each visit, when they leave a way to keep up with that record is you have them sign their card so they sign for the session. Now, they've already paid, but the act of having them sign for that session prior to leaving adds another level of VIP Executive Platinum importance. And it allows the client to see the progression, see how they're building miles, how they're building hours, because they see their signature five times, and ten times, and 15 times, and now they see it 17 times and they only have three left and this is when you, the business person, successful massage practitioner, say to them 'wow you've had 17 sessions you're coming up. Would you like to renew your account before you reach 20' and just go ahead and get that out of the way?

So, it can be used as a tool to help you remind them that it's time for an additional re-up. And the Signature Card, the whole signing process should be done where it's easy and smooth and what that means is invest in very good writing instruments. And you can go to Office Depot, Office Max, and buy good pens. Get the pens that have gel ink because they write very smooth. Get the gel ink pens. Have one in black. Have in blue. You might have one in – I use one in purple because purple looks very regal and make sure you have pens that write really well and smooth and invest in, you can get this at the office place too, invest in one of those nice faux leather clipboards that has a nice little wrist pad on the end and it has a pen holder at the top that I typically just open for them so they can select the pen and then you present them with the writing tablet where they can sign their card and/or write you a check.

When people are being asked to give you money, to write you a check, make sure it is an excellent experience for them. Pens that don't write, pens that are cheap, cheapen the event and tell the person that you really don't care enough to pay attention to the detail like that. Go to any bank and try to write something at the island in the bank with the cheap pens. I have never understood, this is a bank, I am writing out money to give to you and you got a pen that barely will write on a cheap chain that's usually broken or some kid's been chewing on it. It drives me crazy. I mean no wonder Bank of America's in trouble. They're not paying attention to the details.

Well, it is all in the details. One of the things I really want you to talk about, I mean you've mentioned a couple of things already, but my slogan if you will is that 'everything that touches a client is marketing.' Like all these little things you're talking about, the pen, the paper, the vision that they see of your office, the fact that you're trash can's empty or full, and you've talked about a lot of little special little touches. What are some of the other touches you have in your office that are designed to make clients feel special or that are just going to set you apart and realize, you know, they're paying what might be a premium price but they're getting a high value for it?

Yeah, each person receives a small bottle of cool water prior to their departure. So, they can take that with them, sip on it while they're in their vehicle, and of course they have all the water they would like in the office because I have coolers and this sort of thing, but each person gets a small bottle of water to go. And you can go to Sam's Warehouse, Costco, and buy cases of bottled water pretty inexpensively and it's a pretty good investment.

I also offer and have on the desk when they're departing, I use Trinidad Ginger Mints, which are a hit. Many people look forward to those ginger mints. In the past I've used other types of mint chocolates that are placed on the treatment table that they can consume while they are preparing themselves to get on the table. So, I have ginger mints, I have bottled water that's available to people.

Another rule in my office is that when the client is exiting the office, the office proper, I always walk them to the door and I always open the door for them, male or female. I always open the door for them when they exit and I thank them for their business and I especially make it a point to thank them when they write a check out or if pay in cash. I only take checks or cash. I'm a plastic free zone. I don't take credit cards, debit cards, Sears cards, or insurance cards. I'm a cash business and people don't mind paying cash for a good experience and good service.

So, I open the door, they have their bottled water, they have their ginger mint if they so choose and I thank them. Now when the financial transaction takes place the way that I accept the money or the check is I hold the check with two hands between my thumb and first finger, each corner, with it in front of me I give them a slight bow and I thank them for the check and I borrowed that from Japanese culture.

The times that I have spent in Japan I have always been fascinated by the Japanese culture's commitment to service to each other and to people, so I adopted that from Japanese culture, holding business cards with two hands, slight bow, thank the person for that. So, I do that if they give me a $100 bill and a $20 and a $10, I hold the money in my hands, a slight bow of the head, thank you very much I appreciate this and it makes a difference.

Because think about this how many times have you been in a coffee shop or place where you're getting counter help and they have a tip jar there. And so they fix your yogurt or whatever and you're waiting for them to see you put the dollar in the tip jar and they say nothing to you. They don't say 'thank you, how do you do, have a good day, I appreciate it', nothing. I don't know about you it irritates the heck out of me. So, I'm thinking why bother.

Right.

People want to be acknowledged for their payments, whether you're paying to have your car fixed. Whether you're paying to go to the movie theater, this idea of people accepting money and not acknowledging their gratefulness for it in this economy and with so many people out of work and all, you better learn how to thank people for their business and thank them for writing you a check and thank them for paying you. That just makes me crazy.

I mean I'm trying to do a good thing you know, and those hard-working kids behind the counter whatever, you know, hey here's a little tip there, I get nothing. I get nothing. They just go on to the next person, next, okay well appreciate it. Yeah, we notice that kind of stuff. So anyway. . .

No, that's great. Benny with all of your success would you say that you've ever made any marketing mistakes?

Yes, buying print marketing. Okay, forget about newspaper ads, forget about Yellow Page ads, especially now in this time with the Internet. Who's even looking at the Yellow Pages?

Right.

Anybody trying to sell you a Yellow Page ad they've been asleep for 30 years or something. So, yeah, I did print ads, and newspaper, Yellow Pages, buying them in local magazines, none if it ever got me a client in all the years I did it. In the end it was word of mouth because people had a good experience.

Right.

So give people a good experience and that's your best marketing right there. Give them a good experience. Treat that person like they're the only client you have because when you're starting out it could be the only client you have and then you

113

build on that. Make a good experience, you know, start on time, finish on time.

Finishing on time is equally important because people have busy schedules, they have other places to go, they got things to do and contrary to popular belief not everybody wants to lie on the table for five hours and getting a massage because we may think it's great. They got other appointments, other things and so they appreciate it when you get them out on time. So, starting on time is important, but getting them out on time is equally important. They've got to go to the airport; they've got to pick up their kid from school.

And so what do you do if someone shows up late because it happens, you know traffic, accidents, things like that. You still stay within the time that they have purchased. You don't go over the next client's time because that person was unfortunately late, because as soon as you do that you are now training that client to be late. Train your clients to be one time and let me tell you how well I've trained my clients.

I would venture to say that 85% of my clients show up 15 – 25 minutes early for their appointments because they simply enjoy being in that office. They sit in the reading area, see what the latest magazines are, listen to the great music I'm playing, they feel comfortable in there. I may be one of the few businesses where people show up that early and I think some actually show up early because they figure if I start a little early they'll get a little extra, so that's all good. But I've trained them to be on time is my point.

So, as soon as you start doing things like well so and so, client A is 15 minutes late, but I want to give them an hour, so I now go into client B's time, now client B is having to wait, client B is not happy, but then you go over the time but client B had to be at the airport at a certain time and it squeezes him. And I learned these things the hard way. I didn't come straight out understanding this. I mean I made bad mistakes and bad decisions about timing in my early part of my career until I got it so everything that I'm sharing with you has come about because I had to learn the hard way. So, when I started running into other people's time and when I started letting people be late and not making any big deal about it, yeah I got into trouble. So, now I've got everybody trained to be on time because they know I'll be ready for them and they know I'll get them out on time.

Excellent. Any other advice that you could share just in relation to building a practice or being successful. What was it you said yesterday, you called it professional self-esteem. Anything else you'd like to add on that before we close?

Yeah, professional self-esteem, the way you maintain and gain professional self-esteem you should go to massage conferences, conventions, you should take massage therapy continuing education so you can be inspired, so you're creativity can be inspired, so that you can have a networking opportunities and collaborate with your colleagues in other parts of the country and the world with ideas that can be helpful and useful to you if you adopt them. As well as an exchange of good information to save us all time to get to point B.

So professional self-esteem is driven by continuing one's education, whether you're reading books, magazine articles, taking workshops, talking and collaborating with other massage therapists in the area, having local meetings to discuss various types of cases, those things build your professional self-esteem so that you are comfortable with your skills and your knowledge to know when to refer, when not to do and to have professional self-esteem where others in healthcare and wellness will turn to you and send referrals because they feel from you, they see from you and they've heard about you from successful clients you've seen that here's someone that could help you with this challenge that you're having.

And by building and maintaining one's professional self-esteem through continuing education and stimulating your creative side you will then have nourishment for your soul because education nourishes the soul.

Thank you Benny, for a fantastic interview. It has been very insightful!

"Simple and plain things can touch your heart very easily! If you can be simple and plain, you can touch every heart!"
— **Mehmet Murat ildan**

DOWNLOAD YOUR FREE RESOURCES!

Go to www.CreatingLifetimeClients.com and click the tab "Free Resources" to download the FREE Resources from the book – no promo code needed! You'll get full-sized worksheets with all the exercises included in the book that you can print and use again and again as your business grows and changes. Download now so you can use as you read!

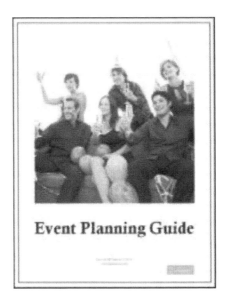

As a bonus, I'm also including several additional special offers and discounts from massage and spa industry companies and organizations PLUS a **FREE Event Planning Guide** – perfect for organizing events and promotions!

Events created without careful planning are not likely to bring in many visitors, generate media interest or add extra sales. This detailed guide will help you prepare for many successful events in your business. Enjoy!

OTHER PRODUCTS

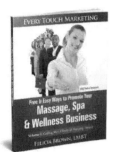

Learn how to get (& keep) clients easily, effectively... and affordably with this new pint-sized power house of a book just for massage, spa and wellness professionals!

Each chapter and strategy in **Free & Easy Ways to Promote Your Massage, Spa & Wellness Business: Volume 1 - Getting New Clients (& Keeping Them!)** will help you move closer to achieving the vision you have for your practice, clinic, or business; connect with and keep your ideal clients; and create a profitable business.

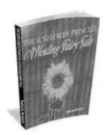

The Sunflower Princess: A Healing Fairy Tale tells a lyrical story about a little seed that has been unexpectedly swept away from her familiar world into one of difficult times and isolation. Through her journey, she learns to have hope and, eventually, "to grow and bloom like no other."
Described by one reader as "a wonderful tool to achieve harmony within" and "a thoughtful & magical gift for a friend or family member in need of meaningful healing" this book was written with adults in mind, but is totally appropriate for children of all ages.

All of the meditations on this CD are original, but they have been inspired by the words and work of many including Louise Hay, Caroline Myss, Wayne Dyer, Marianne Williamson and Shakti Gawain and by my thousands of students and clients. I hope you will use **Just Breathe** with your own clients and students. It is perfect as a pre-treatment relaxation in massage therapy sessions and nail treatments, a meditative add-on during facial or body masks or an end of yoga class cool down.

Order at www.Spalutions.com or www.EveryTouchMarketing.com. Use the Promo Code "LIFETIME" to save 10% on your next order

SPECIAL OFFER - ISLAND SOFTWARE

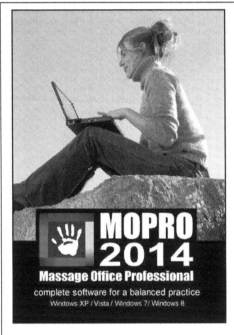

SPECIAL OFFER - CLINIC SENSE SOFTWARE

Get a FREE trial and save $75 on GROW & PRO plans - This practice management software is loved by thousands of solo massage therapy practitioners and small clinics. Just go to https://clinicsense.com/spalutions to get the FREE trial and savings!

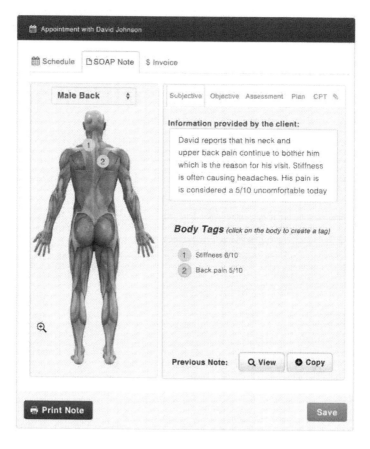

ABOUT THE AUTHOR

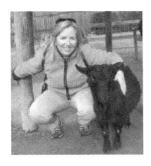

Felicia Brown, LMBT is the owner of Spa*lutions!*, (www.spalutions.com) and provides business and marketing coaching for massage, spa and wellness professionals. She is passionate about inspiring others and has a personal philosophy and practice of sharing her knowledge and experience with others so they may become successful in all of their endeavors. Felicia's practice of "cooperative competition" has been a cornerstone of her career since becoming a massage therapist in 1994.

Felicia has won many awards for her business acumen and industry involvement including: **2014 Best Massage Therapist of the Triad**; **2011 Volunteer of the Year** (*American Massage Conference*); **2009 Spa Person of the Year** (*Day Spa Association*); **2005 Small Business Person of the Year** (*Greensboro Chamber of Commerce*); **Top Entrepreneurs of 2009/Top 25 Movers & Shakers of 2008** (*Business Leader Magazine*), **2007 National Volunteer Committee of the Year** (*American Massage Therapy Association*), **2004 Women in Business** (*The Business Journal*); & **2003 Forty Leaders Under Forty** (*The Business Journal*).

This is Felicia's fourth book. Since her first book came out, she has also published *Reflections of My Heart: A Poetic Journey of Love, Life, Heartbreak and Healing* and *The Sunflower Princess: A Healing Fairy Tale*. Also, Felicia's blog, www.ZenVersusZin.com documents her journey of exploring sobriety and is the "pre-quel" to her planned book of the same name which is due out in 2016. She has also contributed to a number of industry publications and books.

Felicia makes her home in Greensboro, NC. In her spare time, Felicia is a casually competitive tri-athlete and also enjoys yoga, reading, cooking, travel, and spa/travel adventures of most any sort.

When you touch one thing with deep
awareness, you touch everything.
- Lao Tzu

Made in the USA
Charleston, SC
03 June 2016